MY DIVA DIET

A WOMAN'S LAST DIET BOOK

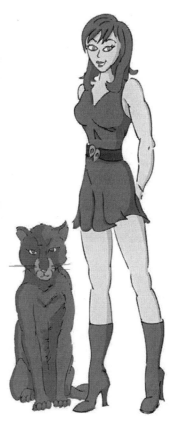

"Hi, I'm Ms. Diva and this is my sidekick Paw—
we are your Fitness Superheroes…

Are YOU ready to attain
a lean, healthy, fit, and more
functional body—for life?"

Created and written by Christine Lakatos

Amber Garman • contributing author

Brian Anderson • web design & creative director

Scott Martin • illustration & book layout and design

Angelica Lakatos • character development

Nicole Stuiber • contributing writer

Michelle Ahearn • contributing editor

Dan Port • contributing editor

Sean Troeger • photography

H. David Segal, M.D. • DIVA web theme song

Disclaimer

This publication expresses the opinions and ideas of its authors. Its purpose is to provide educational information on the subjects addressed herein, and in no way is its content, either implicitly or explicitly, to be interpreted as medical advice or any other personal professional service. MY DIVA DIET was designed to help women lose fat and gain health. It is for women who do not have medical condition(s) requiring a special diet program or medical supervision. Readers should consult a physician prior to beginning any type of diet or exercise program.

MY DIVA DIET is not in the business of attacking any diet product or program, but we are here to present you with facts as well as our opinions about the fitness industry, the American obesity epidemic, quick-fix diets, fat loss, food products, exercise, and other areas related to getting fit and healthy.

The authors and publisher of MY DIVA DIET specifically disclaim all responsibility for any liability, loss, or risk, personal or otherwise, incurred as a consequence, directly or indirectly, of the use and/or application of any of the contents of this book.

Dedication

To all women who want to take charge
and win the battle for health & fitness:
What does it take WIN?
Knowledge, accountability, courage, discipline and motivation!
To those women who are not afraid of this winning formula and
are willing to do what is needed to live better while inspiring others.

For what is done and learned by one class of women becomes, by virtue their common womanhood, the property of all women.

~ Elizabeth Blackwell

Contents

Contents

Working with thousands of clients for over twenty-five years as a fitness professional, I witnessed some phenomenal results and watched lives change for the better.

I watched a sixty-five-year-old woman who had never exercised a day in her life lose twenty pounds, drop seventeen inches and shed four sizes, all while getting off anti-depressants and lowering her cholesterol level. I also saw a client and friend in her late forties lower her body fat from twenty to ten percent and lose fifteen pounds, while improving her health and transforming her body to that of a fit teenager. Another friend in her thirties was an amazing surprise when she dropped her body fat from thirty percent down to a level so low (around fourteen percent) that she had "six-pack abs" and could easily have competed in a fitness competition. Another client in her twenties lived for years with twenty-eight percent body fat and never exercised before she transformed her body (and her life). She now maintains sixteen to eighteen percent body fat year-round.

It's been incredible working with so many women in their fifties, seeing them start off with over thirty-five percent body fat and drop it down to sixteen percent (and keep it off), all while influencing their family and friends to eat better and exercise. Of course many women in their twenties and thirties just wanted a better body—and they got it! I have also trained teenage athletes and watched them get fit while their sports performances improved dramatically.

There have been many radical changes, but also numerous simple ones, that are not less significant. I was honored to work with an eighty-five-year-old cancer patient who weighed only eighty-six pounds. Her workouts led to an increase in muscle and a more positive attitude and she felt much better. It was fun to work with a woman (whose husband was a famous boxer) for only a few sessions, then to see her a few months later and be shocked about how fit she had become. When I asked her what she did to get in such great shape, her response was, "I did what you told me to do".

Another example is when I gave just a little bit of attention and motivation to a young woman who then went on to become Ms. Universe. Even clients that golf were able to build more functional and fit bodies that added distance to their drives and endurance to their games as well as improve their health for life. It's also been a pleasure to be instrumental in decreasing and fixing physical ailments, such as celiac disease, high blood pressure, osteoporosis, heart disease, problems with poor posture and low-back pain, just to name a few (that plagued some clients for years).

Knowing that dieting is a personal topic that is best addressed in a specific format and thus is difficult to generalize, I wanted to design a book that would fit the diet needs of all women, from teenagers to college students to mothers and even to women in their sixties—any woman who wants to lose a few pounds, become more healthy and fit, or experience a major transformation. So the true challenge in designing MY DIVA DIET was this: how can I write a diet book in general terms; meet specific needs and challenges; address a diverse group of women; and still make it inviting, motivating and useful at the same time?

I completely understand the complexity involved in this endeavor. However, my experience in dealing with women of different needs, desires, backgrounds, lifestyles, tastes, interests, as well as varying levels of fitness, awareness, and commitment is precisely why I was able to create a complete, proven and practical fat-loss system.

But there was still one missing link. I began a personal quest to try to answer some of life's basic questions. Why are we here? What is life about? What is my purpose? Throughout my four-year inductive study of scripture (the Bible) I found more than I bargained for. Not only did I discover redemption, morality and true character development, but also I learned that God sheds light not only on his desire for us to be fit and healthy, but also how we can achieve it! I realized that God, the Creator, was our first "trainer" in health and wellness. He teaches us what we should and should not eat and even how to handle, slaughter and prepare animal meat. He is the Creator of women and the designer of food and I trust His Word is true.

From the garden in which we were vegetarians, to after the flood when we began eating both plant and animal foods, to the laws given to the people of Israel and followed by Jesus, the holy scriptures gives us history and directions about diet. It discusses, give lessons and sets examples regarding many other topics like exercise, alcohol, water, portion control, times to be a vegetarian, fasting, preservatives, bread, milk, and much more.

I then incorporated these principles of eating into the MY DIVA DIET program. So whether one believes in God or nature, there is no denying that God's way of eating and what nature produces are:

- Beneficial to health & fitness
- Meant to produce a more peaceful, joyous, abundant and longer life
- Increases energy and productivity
- Better tasting
- Safer
- More humane
- Better for our environment
- More prosperous for our country

MY DIVA DIET was developed through experience and education in the fitness industry, personal application and also anchored in Judeo-Christian principles. Combining experience, knowledge and faith creates a comprehensive diet system just for women–and it works.

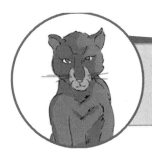

The truth is out there, whether you want to improve your physical or spiritual condition. So pursue TRUTH and you will be amazed at the power it has to transform your life and the lives of others."

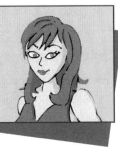

"Don't be afraid of the truth; whether it's for you or against you, honesty leads us to change!"

Christine Lakatos
ACE Certified Fitness Trainer
Creator of MY DIVA DIET
June 2008

Acknowledgements

First I would like to acknowledge that without being a Christian, I never would have found the right path and discipline to succeed at anything that is GOOD! I would like to thank my wonderful daughters, Nicole and Angelica, for their love and patience. To Sister Theresa and Monsignor Rice who were truly my mentors and heroes when I was growing up. To my grandmother, rest her soul, for her constant encouragement and for saying "Christina, you can move mountains". To my sister, Diane, for "being my resucer" over the years—you are terrific! To Mr. Wilson, my childhood track coach, who gave me confidence and who first taught me that "you are what you eat". To Paula Anderson who gave me my start as a fitness competitor and professional. A special thanks to Cynthia Silkenson who truly believed in me and motivated me to write this book. To all my clients along the way who trusted me, did what I told them to do, got results and, at times, shocked me on how this diet works. To all my loving pets who never left my side no matter what!

Last but not least, thanks to my wonderful team, without whom my vision would have never come alive. To Amber Garman, whose help and dedication is so much appreciated. Amber, you truly are an inspiration! Brian Anderson and Scott Martin, who put up with my creativity and insanity and whose talents and expertise made this project better than I ever imagined. To Sean Troeger, my photographer; Michelle Ahearn and Dan Port, my talented editors, for their work. Finally, to our very own neurosurgeon, Dr. Segal, for composing and recording the DIVA web theme song.
~Christine Lakatos

I would also like to greatly acknowledge the entire MY DIVA DIET team. As my aunt and I learned halfway through writing this book, it takes a collection of expertise to complete almost any book. I would also like to thank my parents for their words of motivation and praise, especially my mother for passing along the good food-cooking gene! To my aunt "Chris," who hates that I call her this shortened nickname, for asking me for my help and in becoming partners in something we are both so enthusiastic about. Most importantly, I would like to praise the Lord, for ultimately providing me with the opportunity to endure this experience.
~Amber Garman

Foreword

"I would highly recommend MY DIVA DIET to anyone who wants to obtain a healthy lifestyle and a great-looking body. I am 53 years young, 5'6" and weigh 111 with 14% body fat. Christine taught me that looking good and being healthy is a way of life! Prior to working with Christine there was endless array of trainers and nutritionists that put me on restricted diets and sold me on expensive vitamins that ended up just making me sick. Now I am healthy, vibrant and full of life. I never feel hungry and I know that not only do I look my best, but I have enough energy to get me through the day and yet fall asleep peacefully at night. Christine really knows nutrition and health! She also looks fantastic! What a great role model she has been for me! Her approach is so reasonable and yet so unique in this world of trendy diets and gimmicks. This is truly the last diet book you will ever read. It works and it is something I can stick with because it is about living a healthy and clean life.

Many thanks to My Diva Christine Lakatos for giving me the body I always wanted and giving me the tools for living a healthy life!
  ~Cynthia Silkensen

PART ONE

The Introduction

Become the change you want to see
—those are the words I live by.
~ Oprah Winfrey

MY DIVA DIET Philosophy

Ms. Diva Asks, "Do You Know . . . ?" *

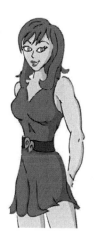

- Americans shell out some $50 billion on weight-loss products each year. Yet we are still fat!
- Half of us are overweight—and 31 to 38% of our children are obese.
- It's estimated that at least 29% of all Americans (and 50% of U.S. women) are on a diet.
- Of the 50 million Americans who attempt a diet program, only 5 to 10% succeed.
- 95% of dieters will regain their lost weight in one to five years.
- Millions still succumb to "quick-fix" claims, seeking a (non-existent) effortless weight-loss method.
- Most fashion models are thinner than 98% of American women.
- Four out of five women say they're dissatisfied with the way they look.
- 91% of college women have attempted to control their weight by dieting often or continuously.
- Almost 50% of children ages six to eight say they want to be thinner.
- Four out of five ten-year-old girls are afraid of being fat and 50% of nine and ten-year-old girls say that being on a diet makes them feel better about themselves.
- It is estimated that 5 to 10% of American women and teenage girls (i.e., 5 to 10 million) are struggling with eating disorders.
- Eating disorders affect three times as many people as does schizophrenia and AIDS.
- During one person's lifetime, 50,000 people will die as a direct result of eating disorders.

---

* Sources
- Bankrate.com (story by Ellen Goodstein)
- Calorie Control Council (caloriecontrol.org)
- CBS News, "Diet Industry Is Big Business" (story by Sharon Alfonsi)
- HealthyWithin.com (statistics and pre-signs of eating disorders)
- INCH-A-WEIGH.COM
- NEDIC (National Eating Disorder Information Center) news
- Penn State University Health Services

The average American woman is about 32% body fat, which medically is considered obese. The average American woman is a size fourteen and experiences a variety of premature medical conditions.

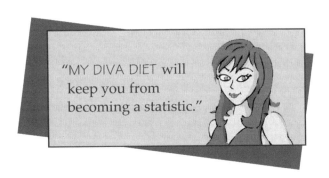

"MY DIVA DIET will keep you from becoming a statistic."

We need to confront the fact that poor nutrition and lack of exercise usually trigger our weight difficulties as well as some of the medical predicaments we find ourselves facing. However, the methods we use to confront these issues are extreme, to say the least. Instead of trying to gain control over our diet problem the right way, we have become desperate, seeking out programs that only end up as major disappointments—creating multiple health risks and costing us money.

We women can stop all the confusion and even help the next generation of girls and young women. Instead of settling for our current condition and seeking a quick-fix product or program, we can get healthy & fit once and for all the right way by searching for accurate knowledge and by disciplining ourselves.

MY DIVA DIET: For Women Only

You are about to begin learning about a very direct approach to dieting. We are not interested in attacking any product or program but instead are here to teach you the truth. You will be the judge of any program or product on your own. We are not here to sell false promises, gimmicks, special pills, or potions. We have already figured out that there is no quick fix to losing fat—but we do know it is possible.

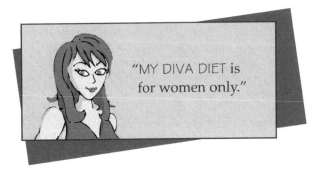

"MY DIVA DIET is for women only."

The MY DIVA DIET program is designed for women only and mainly for those women who do not have a medical condition that requires a special diet program or medical supervision. Consult with your doctor!

4

The MY DIVA DIET mission is to help women of all ages (from teenagers to healthy women over sixty) reach a very attractive and obtainable body fat level (25% or less), while maintaining and/or improving health.

MY DIVA DIET is equally effective for women who want to lose five and even up to fifty pounds and more. We can take a woman with 40% body fat and get her down to 30% or less. We can also take a lean woman at 19% body fat and bring her down to 15%. Whatever your desire and commitment level, we can help you lose fat!

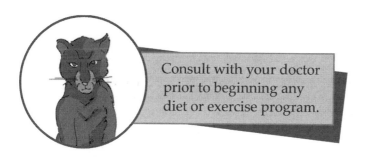

Consult with your doctor prior to beginning any diet or exercise program.

What makes MY DIVA DIET so special? Well, besides the fact that it works, it is based on a lifestyle change: not only do you lose body fat and improve your health, but you will also be able to maintain the results you worked so hard to achieve.

MY DIVA DIET is designed to help you lose those unwanted fat pounds (and cellulite) without sacrificing your health or sanity. No responsible diet will ever compromise your physical or mental health for the sake of looking good. Health & fitness should always work synergistically. In fact, as you get into shape you will automatically improve your overall health and mental well-being.

MY DIVA DIET is not about suffering or starving. It is not full of distress or pain. It does not promote confusion or desperation. But MY DIVA DIET is not a program of "anything goes" either—it does have some boundaries. MY DIVA DIET is not about denying food but rather understanding food and embracing it as your friend. It is about a lifestlye of proper eating and exercise that will get you the body you've always dreamed and newfound energy—for life!

The Core of MY DIVA DIET

The central and most important part of the MY DIVA DIET program is the quality of the foods that we advocate for losing fat, improving health, and staying fit for the rest of your life. See our Paw Guide below:

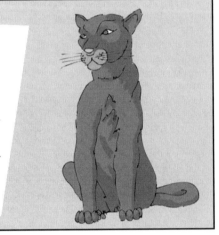

Paw Food Guide

- Clean and pure foods—natural, fresh, organic, and kosher
- Lean, healthy, fibrous, and *alive* foods
- Foods made by God (nature) for human consumption
- Carefully chosen man-made or man-manipulated foods

MY DIVA DIET advocates wholesome foods. Foods that promote mental, spritual and physical well-being. Foods that are made by God (nature) and intended for human consumption. And, MY DIVA DIET is very selective in its recommendations of foods made or manipulated by man.

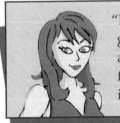

"It is interesting to note that man can go to the moon, cure many diseases, and accomplish other extraordinary feats, but when man alters food from its natural state, he usually ruins it."

MY DIVA DIET Food Criteria

MY DIVA DIET has designed two valuable diet tools, found in PART TWO (the Diva Reduction Pyramid on page 31 and the Diva Maintenance Pyramid on page 46). Each tool summarizes MY DIVA DIET food standards in a single page.

Throughout this workbook you will also find many other useful special designs, guides, tips, charts, and diet tools that will help you succeed in your goals for fat loss and better health.

What We Offer

* FIRST (and foremost): MY DIVA DIET addresses the root causes of why we are overweight and not at our full potential for optimal health. These comprise the Five Factors Affecting Body Fat and Health. To help you understand how these factors work for or against you, you will be taking a diet quiz in PART THREE (pages 61-83) for specific answers about why you are in shape—or not.

* SECOND: We believe that all women are created equal, but we are also unique and we have distinct needs even in the world of dieting. Because MY DIVA DIET is designed specifically for women, it focuses on women's concerns ranging from our frame sizes and body weight to our health & fitness goals to our hectic schedules.

* THIRD: The MY DIVA DIET workbook is interactive and user-friendly. We have created this more personal approach to dieting because we want you to get involved in the process. Your active participation will help you learn more, stay encouraged and become more empowered in accomplishing your goals.
  - You will find your own workspace in PART EIGHT (pages 327-386), where you will learn about body fat and how it is measured. You can set goals for body fat, measurements and size in order to track your goals for your anticipated progress.
  - You can track your food intake as well as your daily intake of protein, carbohydrates, fat, fiber, and sodium. You can even calculate your nutrient ratio.
  - We give you a personal calendar to track your diet and exercise.
  - Finally, there are many worksheets and your own personal journal pages to write down questions, concerns, comments, and feelings.

By using this methodical approach to dieting and by actively exploring the root causes of weight gain, you will most definitely stay on course and achieve your goals for a leaner, more functional, healthier body. You may even resolve some health issues you have battled for many years. You will feel and look better than you ever have—and you may even enjoy the ride along the way!

Use this nameplate to make this workbook yours now:

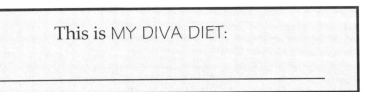

This is MY DIVA DIET:

_____

Warning: Using this workbook requires commitment. It is best to follow the MY DIVA DIET program for at least ten weeks or longer to truly get the results you desire.

This type of commitment will enable you to ultimately change your eating habits for life so that you will keep the fat off and stay healthy for the rest of your life. Whatever you do to achieve your goal of fat loss and optimal health, you will need to continue to make at least 65% to 75% of that effort to maintain your results.

* FOURTH: MY DIVA DIET provides you with multiple tools for success:
  - How to recognize your true Diet Villains
  - Information on the difference between fat loss and weight loss
  - An accurate analysis of your current condition via the Diva 32-Question Diet Quiz, with notes and rules on how to address each of the sub-topics within the Five Factors
  - How to lose fat and maintain your low body fat
  - Menu plan (meals and recipes) and diet cheating for fat loss
  - Lists and charts on what to eat, when to eat, and how much to eat
  - Information on calories, fiber and food products
  - Information on reading labels and how to test foods for health & fitness
  - Guides on grocery shopping, food preperation and cooking, restaurant eating, and much more

* FIFTH: MY DIVA DIET is a program based on sound nutrition and backed by more than twenty-five years of knowledge and experience in the fitness industry. Our experience in the fitness industry provides us with the ability necessary to design a power packed and practical diet book! We are excited about sharing our expertise with you and your family.

Our genuine hope is that we women will *not* leave our children a legacy of ignorance in the field of diet and exercise. MY DIVA DIET wants to give you the information you need to begin setting healthful patterns for your families. We want you to motivate and educate the next generation so that unhealthy habits can be eradicated once and for all.

✳ SIXTH: MY DIVA DIET has developed a unique approach to help you learn about healthy eating and visualize how much power you really have in your battle against fat. Our Superheroes—Ms. Diva and her sidekick, Paw—will teach and coach you through the entire MY DIVA DIET program and encourage you to take charge of your bodies as you wage war against your true diet enemies.

"We don't ever want you to forget us—
or the information we offer."

The Five Factors Affecting Body Fat and Health

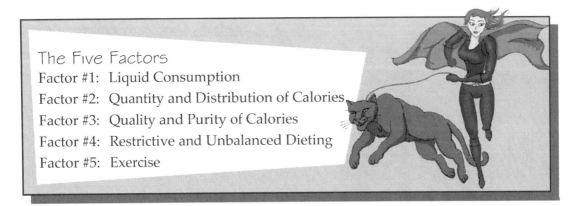

The Five Factors
Factor #1: Liquid Consumption
Factor #2: Quantity and Distribution of Calories
Factor #3: Quality and Purity of Calories
Factor #4: Restrictive and Unbalanced Dieting
Factor #5: Exercise

Before we go any further, it is very important that you become familiar with the Five Factors Affecting Body Fat and Health. This summary will be your guide to eating for the rest of your life. Knowing and understanding these factors is crucial to your fat loss and improved health success.

Factor #1: Liquid Consumption
Too many poor liquid choices add unnecessary and empty calories to the American diet, and an inadequate water intake leaves women dehydrated, unhealthy, and unhappy.

Factor #2: Quantity and Distribution of Calories
- Daily caloric intake (uncontrolled calories—too many or not enough)
- Daily nutrient ratio: protein/carbohydrates/fat (unbalanced calories)
- Number of meals in each day (too many or not enough)
- Meal size (uncontrolled portions)
- Meal timing (unmonitored timing)

Factor #3: Quality and Purity of Calories
- Fat calories
- Unhealthy calories
- Dirty calories

- Impure calories
- Old and dead calories
- Non-kosher calories

Factor #4: Restrictive and Unbalanced Dieting

Because most women look for quick-fix solutions to our obesity and poor-health epidemic, we buy into gimmicks and false promises. We subscribe to dangerous pills and special packaged foods. We suffer needlessly. Sometimes we lose weight only to "rebound"—gaining more weight than when we started and usually at the expense of our health. We end up confused and more desperate. So instead of seeking the proper way to lose weight, we start the cycle all over again.

Factor #5: Exercise

Lack of exercise is a major factor in our health and often explains why we may be fat in the first place. We are a "remote-control" country: we lack physical activity and are frequently too lazy to exercise.

How MY DIVA DIET Addresses the Five Factors

The secret to MY DIVA DIET is that we dissect these Five Factors and put together a comprehensive plan to ensure that calories are used for their intended purpose—energy and health.

Factor #1: Liquid consumption is monitored.

Factor #2: The quantity and distribution of calories are calculated.

- Total daily calories are approximately 1,200 to 1,600 (or more in some instances, depending on whether you are in the Diva Reduction Phase or Diva Maintenance Phase of MY DIVA DIET, your activity level, and other variables).
- Daily nutrient ratio for fat loss is 35% protein/45% carbs/20% fat (or close) and approximately 20 to 35% protein/45 to 65% carbs/20 to 30% for maintenance.
- Number of meals is four to five per day.
- Meal sizes are controlled appropriately (portion control).
- Meals are timed appropriately (every three to four hours).

Factor #3: The quality and purity of calories are determined.
- They must be lean (containing little or no fat, especially bad fat).
- They must be healthy (conducive to health).
- They must be clean (free from foreign or extraneous matter).
- They must be pure (free from contamination).
- They must be alive and/or fresh (recently harvested, with no decay, not preserved or processed, and not overcooked)
- They should be kosher (fit and suitable).

Factor #4: Restrictive and unbalanced dieting is eliminated forever.

Factor #5: Exercise is introduced in a balanced regimen.
An effective exercise program should include:
- Cardiovascular conditioning
- Strength and endurance training
- Flexibility training
- Core and balance training
- Corrective exercises
- Functional training

Meet Your Fitness Superheroes

Meet your fitness superheroes, Ms. Diva & Paw and learn their story.

At the dawn of the 21st century, the Diet Villains have reached the highest levels of power. With promises of fatter wallets, they have overtaken the food industry, saturating the market with unhealthy processed foods and man-made products that have nearly squashed the nurturing effects of a natural diet. Their success seems inevitable.

Meanwhile, small-town organic vegetable farmer Crystal Hannah experiences an epiphany after a long day at her local farmer's market. On the drive home, she is bombarded by advertisements for fast foods, fatty treats, and quick fix diets that make absurd promises, but can be severely detrimental to one's health. The evidence of the Diet Villains' influence in our country is all around us and Crystal is seeing it clearly.

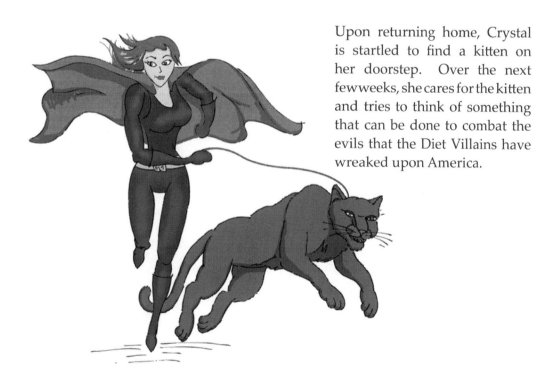

Upon returning home, Crystal is startled to find a kitten on her doorstep. Over the next few weeks, she cares for the kitten and tries to think of something that can be done to combat the evils that the Diet Villains have wreaked upon America.

The kitten grows bigger and bigger, and finally Crystal awakens one day to see that the kitten has actually grown into a mighty panther. Even more shocking, the panther speaks to her and introduces himself as Paw. He tells her that through her care for her body, mind, spirit, and her organic farm, she has proven herself to be a strong-willed and caring individual who is capable of taking on the Diet Villains and helping women everywhere take steps toward a healthy and fulfilling lifestyle of diet and exercise. The revolution for women everywhere is to begin, and she is to be the one to lead it.

Crystal is initially fearful, but she is determined to help women everywhere find fitness, health, and happiness, and she accepts the challenge. Paw then puts her through a rigorous physical conditioning program. When she has completed her training, Crystal is equipped with the physical strength and stamina, and has developed the courage, knowledge, and discipline she needs for her mission. As part of her transformation, she is given special superhero powers (found in her belt) to restrain the evil of the Diet Villains.

With Paw's help, she creates a plan for women everywhere and of all ages and types. She also adopts the persona of Ms. Diva, a proud woman of forceful temperament who will stand up to the Diet Villains.

And so Ms. Diva and her sidekick Paw are set to take on all of the Diet Villains and vanquish them forever.

Ms. Diva's message to you is simple and direct:

"We are in a battle for our health & fitness, and in any battle we should know our enemies! Together we can stop the confusion and expose, attack, and defeat the Diet Villains. You can help Paw and I conquer these malicious villains in your life and the lives of others!"

Know Your Diet Villains

Know the roles that the Diet Villains play in the Five Factors.

Factor #1: Liquid Consumption

POPS: Dehydration from drinking too little water and too many bad fluids like soda and other sugary drinks

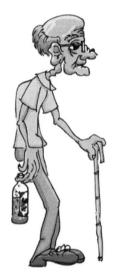

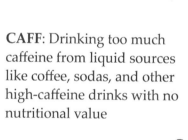

CAFF: Drinking too much caffeine from liquid sources like coffee, sodas, and other high-caffeine drinks with no nutritional value

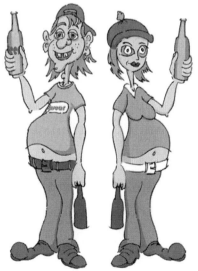

AL and his twin sister, **COLE**: Drinking too much alcohol

Factor #2: Quantity and Distribution of Calories
(Overeating and Undereating)

JOE STUFFT: Overeating

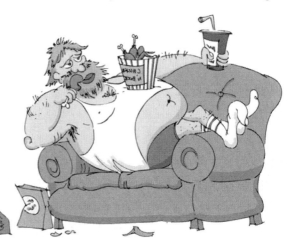

GIRLIE DIE AND HER POODLE, IT: Undereating and other food-disorders like excessive dieting, starvation, pill-taking, etc.

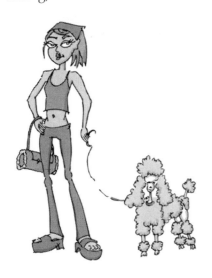

Factor #3: Quality and Purity of Calories (Fat, Unhealthy, Dirty, Impure, Old and Dead, and Non-Kosher Calories)

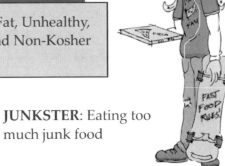

JUNKSTER: Eating too much junk food

16

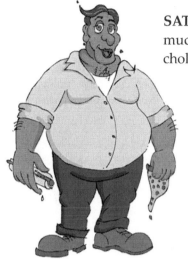

SAT FAT: Consuming too much saturated fat and cholesterol

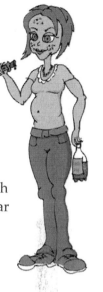

SHOOG: Using too much sugar and too many sugar derivatives and sugar substitutes

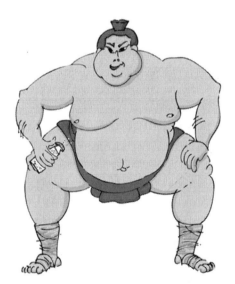

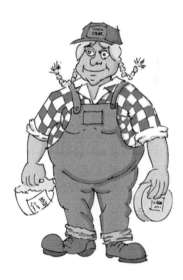

SODI SUMO: Using too much sodium (salt and sodium derivatives)

DAIRY MAIDEN: Consuming too many dairy products (milk, cheese, ice cream, butter, etc.)—especially non-organic

17

TRANNY GRANNY:
Consuming trans fats, hydrogenated oils, and other harmful preservatives and additives

MR. BAKERMAN: Using and overusing white flour and other baking ingredients like starch, baking powder, and dextrin. And, consuming too many baked goods like cookies, donuts, pies, and cakes.

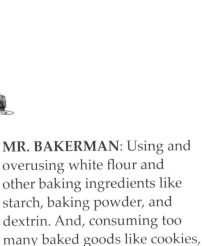

MRS. REGRET: Suffering from an unknown illness caused by all the pesticides, hormones, and antibiotics she has ingested. She constantly moans, "I wish I had eaten natural, fresh, organic, and kosher foods!"

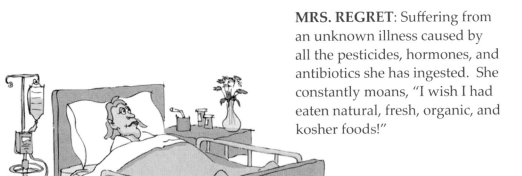

Factor #4: Restrictive and Unbalanced Dieting

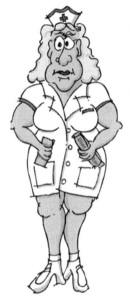

NURSE GIMMICK:
Using every "quick-fix"
diet plan and gimmick
weight-loss diet book,
program, and product

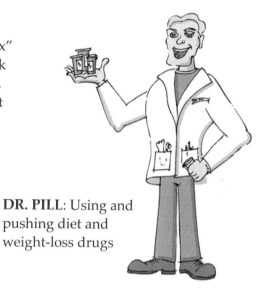

DR. PILL: Using and
pushing diet and
weight-loss drugs

Factor #5: Exercise

VEGG: Avoiding exercise, always
inactive and lazy

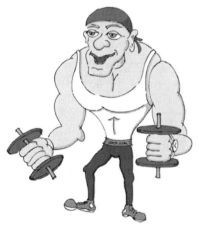

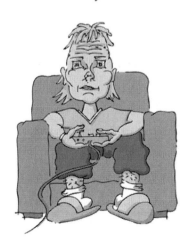

GEORGE GOTTA GO: Exercising obsessively,
using steroids and other performance-enhancing
drugs, and abusing so-called "body-altering"
drugs, whether synthetic or natural

19

MY DIVA DIET Program Overview

What makes MY DIVA DIET unique is that it is a general program for all women that can be individualized for every woman. It is divided into Phase One—Diva Reduction and Phase Two—Diva Maintenance.

What gives MY DIVA DIET its power is that we address the root causes of why women are fat and unhealthy in the first place, and we help you address them once and for all. We also expose the truth about the adversaries you will be facing—i.e., the Diet Villains (pages 15-19)—as you create a new and healthier lifestyle.

This complete program and plan of action will help you achieve your optimal fitness and health levels—as well as look and feel great!

Paw Guide to Using MY DIVA DIET – 7 Ways

#1: Follow the entire program strictly for 6 to 10 weeks for a major transformation in body fat and health.

#2: Follow the entire program semi-strictly for just a few weeks to lose weight and improve your health.

#3: Follow 50 to 70% of the entire program for any time frame to make progress with your body fat and health.

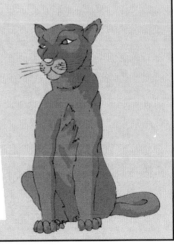

#4: Fix just one of the Five Factors Affecting Body Fat and Health to lose weight and improve your health.

#5: Read the workbook to learn better ways of eating, effective exercise programs, and much more.

#6: Use the workbook as a guide to teach your children healthy ways of eating so they won't fall victim to the deception of the Diet Villains.

#7: Use as a tool to prevent obesity and poor health.

Whatever your goals are, you will benefit in any number of ways, whether you want to go all the way with a major body transformation or just learn to eat better.

What Is Diet Anyway?

"Diet" is not a bad four-letter word: it is defined as the food a person usually consumes or a controlled intake of food and drink designed for weight loss, for health or religious reasons, or to control a medical condition. Don't be afraid of this word in the MY DIVA DIET name—we are just trying to form a new lifestyle involving changes in our food consumption.

An Individualized Program

As you begin the MY DIVA DIET program, it is vital for you to understand that losing fat and improving health are individual objectives. There are many variables that can affect your progress. Three main ones are:

- Your beginning condition (body fat level and health)
- Your goals
- Your commitment level

Other considerations are your lifestyle, age, level of fitness, special health issues, medications you might be taking, etc.

How Much Weight Can You Lose on MY DIVA DIET and How Fast?

When you start a diet program to achieve fat loss, you want results. MY DIVA DIET wants fitness results for you too, but we want to help you reach them in the safest and most effective way possible. As we mentioned earlier, we want you to become fit, but we don't want you to sacrifice your health or your sanity.

You can lose anywhere from five to over fifty pounds on MY DIVA DIET if you want. If you follow the program strictly, you can lose five to ten pounds or more right away. After that, you should plan on losing about one to two pounds per week. Keep in mind that this is a general guide—everyone is different. And—again—your progress is really up to you.

The best part is that by losing fat (not just weight) you can decrease your body fat from 1% to 10%. This fat loss means you will definitely lose anywhere from a few inches around your waist to fifteen inches all over your body. You can reduce your dress size by one or by up to as many as five sizes—for a whole new wardrobe.

Food Sensitivity

Some of you may be aware of food intolerances and food allergies. They are different. We will just call them both "food sensitivities." Both can cause a variety of physical reactions, like water retention, tendency to gain weight, puffiness, abdominal pain, bloating, gas, diarrhea, constipation, hives, itching, nasal congestion, fatigue, mood swings, headaches, and more.

Among the common foods we find ourselves reacting to are cow's milk and dairy products, eggs, wheat, corn and corn products, yeast, soy, sugar, nuts, and shellfish. Some people are even allergic to strawberries.

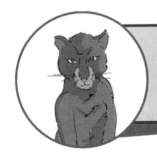

If you know you have a certain allergy or intolerance to any food, then by all means drop it from your diet and be aware of food products that contain these items. If you think you have a specific allergy, consult your doctor or a nutritionist.

Gluten-Free Foods

Gluten is a highly complex protein that occurs in four main grains—wheat, rye, barley and oats—as well as in other grains, including spelt and triticale, so it is present in many products. Gluten-intolerant people find gluten difficult to digest, while others have a more serious reaction called celiac disease. Both problems are more common than you think and can cause many uncomfortable symptoms, including headaches, mouth ulcers, weight gain or loss, poor immunity to disease, skin problems, and other gastrointestinal disorders.

We at MY DIVA DIET advocate a wheat- and flour-free diet in the Diva Reduction Phase and want you to use gluten-free products whenever possible. Wheat and other whole grains are healthy, but it is the overuse and manipulation of these grains that becomes the problem. We also want you to put products made from grains in perspective. You will find that by making these changes in your diet you will change your weight immediately and your health will improve over time.

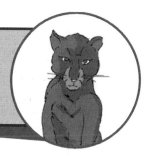

If you know you are gluten-intolerant or have celiac disease, you can follow MY DIVA DIET with special adjustments. If you think you may have these conditions, see your doctor for a proper diagnosis and treatment protocol.

What About Cheating?

We have provided you with a Diva Smart Diet Cheat Sheet in PART FIVE (pages 216-219). Cheating is part of our program, so don't worry. However, when it comes to cheating, less is better. Try not to cheat for the first two weeks. This will help change your tastes and enable you to get a good start on your discipline.

In Phase One—Diva Reduction, keep your choices to the list provided (gluten-free is best) and the portion listed. Cheat only once per week or less.

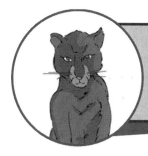

It's always best to cheat on real foods, not on junk food. As your tastes change, soda, hot dogs, fries, donuts, candy, fake foods, white flour, etc., will actually become repellent to you.

In Phase Two—Diva Maintenance, your cheating should still be only once per week from the Diva Smart Diet Cheat Sheet, but in this phase you can add another type of cheating: one to two times per month you can deviate from the program. As you learn more about foods, you can create your own diet cheat sheet.

All-Vegetarian Days

To ensure health and vitality, MY DIVA DIET recommends that you try a once-a-month "all-vegetarian day" during both the Diva Reduction Phase and the Diva Maintenance Phase. Just choose quality fresh fruits, vegetables, whole grains and grain products, legumes, peas, nuts, and seeds for these special days.

Diva 32-Question Diet Quiz—PART THREE (pages 61-83)

We have taken the Five Factors Affecting Body Fat and Health and created the Diva 32-Question Diet Quiz to give you a more personal and comprehensive approach to dieting. The quiz includes grading and tutoring sections so you can analyze each factor individually to see which factors you do (or don't) have under control. You can use this information to facilitate a major transformation, to adjust part of your diet, or just to help you eat better. You can go directly to the quiz now, or you can learn about the Five Factors and the thirty-two sub-topics first.

The following is a quick reference guide on each factor and the relevant areas of dieting for better health and low body fat. This will help those of you who want to learn about specific areas.

Factor #1: Liquid Consumption

1. Water
2. Coffee and other caffeinated drinks
3. Tea
4. Soda
5. Other drinks (sports drinks, powdered soft drinks, juice boxes and other sugary drinks)
6. Juice (fruit and vegetable): fresh vs. concentrated
7. Meal replacement drinks (protein shakes, smoothies and green drinks)
8. Alcohol

Factor #2:   Quantity and Distribution of Calories

9. Daily caloric intake (overeating or undereating)

1,200 to 1,600 depending on phase, activity levels and other variables

- Diva Reduction Phase = 1,200 to 1,300
- Diva Maintenance Phase = 1,400 to 1,600 (or more for certain women)

10. Daily nutrient ratio: protein/carbohydrates/fat
    - Ideal for fat reduction = 35% protein/45% carbs/20% fat
    - Ideal for maintenance = 20 to 35% protein/45 to 65% carbs/20 to 30% fat
11. Number of meals per day (including snacks)
12. Meal timing
13. Meal size (portion control)

Factor #3:   Quality and Purity of Calories
14. Junk food (fast food, pizza, ice cream, potato chips, cookies, candy, donuts, etc.)
15. Total daily fat intake (grams)
16. Total daily sugar intake (grams)
17. Sugar substitutes intake (aspartame, saccharine, Splenda and other artificially made sweeteners)
18. Total daily sodium intake (milligrams)
19. Quality protein intake
20. Quality carbohydrate intake
21. Quality fat intake
22. Total daily dairy intake
23. Clean calories (reading labels/things to look for)
    - Preservatives and additives
    - Flavoring agents, coloring agents, sweeteners (artificial and natural), emulsifiers, texturizers, stabilizers, etc.
    - Chemicals and other fake foods
    - Hidden fats (hydrogenated vegetable oils and other unneeded and unhealthy fats)
    - Hidden sugars (maltodextrin, corn syrup, high fructose corn syrup, etc.)
    - Hidden sodium (salt, MSG, sodium benzoate, sodium nitrate, ferrous sulfate, etc.)
    - Hidden flour (white flour, baking powder, starch, dextrin, etc.)
24. Purity of calories
    - Natural foods vs. processed
    - Fresh foods vs. man-manipulated
    - Organic vs. non-organic
    - Kosher vs. non-kosher

25. White flour intake (bread, cereals, crackers, noodles, pasta, pastries, tortillas, etc.)
26. Total daily fiber intake (grams)
27. Food, sports, energy and protein bars
28. Sauces, salad dressing, dips and condiment intake
29. Cooking and seasoning (fruits, vegetables, herbs, spices)
30. Supplement intake (vitamins, minerals and others)

Factor #4:   Restrictive and Unbalanced Dieting
31. Restrictive and unbalanced diets
   - High-protein, high-fat, no-carbohydrate diets
   - Fruit-only diets
   - Juice-fasting diets
   - Diet pills and liquids
   - And others

Factor #5: Exercise
32. Weekly exercise program
   - Cardiovascular conditioning
   - Strength and endurance training
   - Flexibility training
   - Core and balance training
   - Corrective exercises
   - Functional training

You can complete a more thorough diet analysis in PART EIGHT (Diva Worksheets #3 and #4—pages 356-366) by filling out a food journal and counting your actual intake of calories, protein, carbohydrates, fat, fiber, and sodium. This will give you a clear picture of exactly how many calories per day you are consuming and your nutrient ratio.

In summary, MY DIVA DIET incorporates all Five Factors Affecting Body Fat and Health into one comprehensive diet program that works! Using the thirty-two subtopics listed above, MY DIVA DIET directs you within each of the Five Factors between two phases (Diva Reduction and Diva Maintenance) beginning in PART TWO.   For the best results, read through this material prior to beginning the actual Menu Plan for Fat Loss in PART FIVE (pages 153-181).

However, if you are eager to begin, you can always go directly to PART FIVE and begin the program at any time. Once again, you can get as involved as you want—this is *your* DIVA DIET!

MY DIVA DIET provides everything a woman needs for both short- and long-term fat loss and improved health. With our complete directions, workbook format, special designs, guides, tips and charts, meal options and

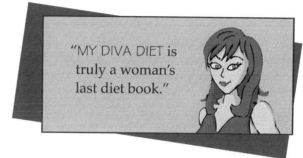

"MY DIVA DIET is truly a woman's last diet book."

recipes, and information about foods, nutrition, exercise, body fat, calories, and more, you will never need to resort to another diet system!

You might add other health and nutrition books, recipes, and ideas to your diet library, but in the future you will know exactly how to analyze any new program, product, or book that comes along.

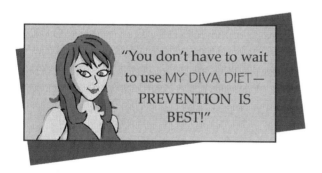

"You don't have to wait to use MY DIVA DIET— PREVENTION IS BEST!"

PART TWO

The Diet

Don't be afraid of things that seem difficult in the beginning. That's only the initial impression. The important thing is not to retreat. You have to master yourself.

~ Olga Korbut

Phase One: Diva Reduction Pyramid

(MY DIVA DIET Food Criteria)

1,200 to 1,300 Calories
Per Day (Average)—For 10 weeks
- 35% protein/45% carbs/20% fat
- 4 to 5 meals per day
- Clean and pure foods
- Natural, fresh, organic, and kosher foods

- High in water intake
- High in nutrients
- High in antioxidants
- High in real/live pure organic foods
- High in alkaline-forming foods (low acidic-forming)
- High in the proper balance of protein, carbs, and fat
- High in fiber

- Alcohol-free
- Flourless/white flour-free
- Wheat-free, partially gluten-free
- Free of artificial ingredients
- Free of genetically modified foods
- Junk food-free

- Extremely low to no processed and refined foods
- Extremely low in food additives and preservatives
- Naturally low-glycemic

- Extra low dairy
- Extra low sugar
- Extra low sodium
- Extra low in saturated fats and cholesterol

Phase One: Diva Reduction—For Ten Weeks

Phase One—Diva Reduction of the MY DIVA DIET program is based on 1,200 to 1,300 calories a day for ten weeks. You may start with three to six weeks if you choose.

The targeted nutrient ratio for Phase One—Diva Reduction is:
- 35% protein/45% carbohydrates/20% fat (those of you who want to be extra-lean Divas can reduce fat intake to 15%).

So, for a 1,300-calorie day, you would eat approximately 113 grams of protein/ 150 grams of carbs/28 grams of fat.

Phase One—Diva Reduction is created as "close to ideal" for dieting. If we adhered to all the dietary rules, we would be a vision of perfection with 13% body fat, lacking many of the common health issues we face today. But we are not perfect; we do not live in an ideal world. MY DIVA DIET takes this into account and also reminds you that some fat on our bodies is not only healthy, but attractive.

As you begin following Phase One, many scenarios may play out:

Case #1: You lose fat at the rate (reasonable, of course) that you want and you are perfectly content. When you reach your goals, you move on to Phase Two— Diva Maintenance.

Case #2: You lose some weight after six weeks. You are happy, but you want to lose more. Continue the diet until you reach your goal (remember: ideally you should sustain the Diva Reduction Phase for ten weeks). Then go on to the Diva Maintenance Phase.

Case #3: You hit a plateau (not at week one or two, but at week five or six). We can offer you some "tricks of the trade," like staggering your calories, changing your meal timing, lowering carbohydrates in certain meals, exercising at a certain time of day, and much more—contact us at www.MyDivaDiet.com.

Case #4: You lose weight too quickly. Just eat more high-quality foods or go directly to the Diva Maintenance Phase.

Case #5: You are already lean (18% body fat) and you want to get leaner—we can help with this too.

Paw Caloric Intake Guide

In the Diva Reduction Phase, it's important to calculate your daily caloric intake so you know how many calories you are consuming each day and how to gauge your daily caloric intake for fat reduction.

Here are some examples:

- If you are consuming 2,000 calories a day, you may only need to drop to between 1,400 and 1,600 per day to reach your goal.
- If you've just come off a restrictive- or starvation-diet plan (1,000 calories per day or less), you may need to slowly build up your daily calories, starting with 1,000 and slowly moving up into the 1,200 to 1,300 range.
- If you exercise regularly or you are an athlete, you may need more than 1,300 calories; even if you are trying to lose fat.

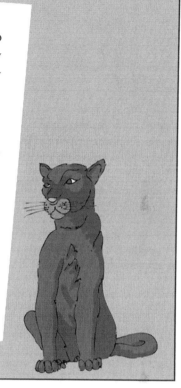

Special Notes:

- For more detailed information on how to calculate your total daily calories, see the 3-Day Diet Analysis in PART EIGHT (pages 356-365).
- As mentioned in PART ONE, you can take the Diva 32-Question Diet Quiz— PART THREE (pages 61-83) at any time to see how your current diet and exercise habits fit into the Five Factors.

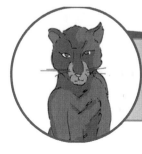

During Phase One, try not to cheat for the first 2 weeks. After that, you can cheat up to once per week, but only from the Diva Smart Diet Cheat Sheet in PART FIVE (pgs. 216-219).

The Five Factors in the Diva Reduction Phase
(Per the Diva 32-Question Diet Quiz—PART THREE, pages 61 to 83)

Factor #1: Liquid Consumption

Water
- Liquids should be limited to water and teas with no sugar. Try to drink approximately six to ten cups of water throughout the day (or more, depending on your body weight, exercise level, current diet, caffeine and alcohol consumption, and any medications you may be taking).

Coffee and other caffeinated drinks
- Coffee is fine, but do not drink high-fat, high-sugar coffee drinks.
- Add some low-fat dairy, soy, or rice milk, and/or a splash of agave nectar or honey in your coffee if you need the flavor.
- Be leery of so called "energy" drinks. They have far too much caffeine and most of them are full of sugar and other unneeded ingredients.

Tea
- Green, red, and black teas are great tea choices.
- Herbal teas are good choices too.

Sodas and other drinks
- Avoid sodas, powdered drinks, juice boxes, fruit drinks, or sports drinks—they are full of sugar.
- Stay clear of drinks labeled as "diet". They contain artificial sweeteners and are not a good idea.

Juices (fruit and vegetable): fresh vs. concentrated
- Juices should be kept to a minimum, and only use fresh-squeezed.

Meal replacement drinks
- Meal replacement drinks like protein shakes, smoothies, and green drinks can be used as substitutes for any meal.
- Ensure the quality of products you use or make them yourself.

Alcohol
- Do not consume alcohol for faster results in Phase One.
- During the Diva Maintenance Phase you can have alcohol in moderation.

Factor #2: Quantity and Distribution of Calories

Daily caloric intake (overeating or undereating)
- The Diva Reduction Phase is based on 1,200 to 1,300 calories per day, ideally for ten weeks. However, start off with three to six weeks and see how much fat you lose, then make adjustments to lose more or go on to the Diva Maintenance Phase.
- This total caloric intake is strict for now but can be adjusted during any part of the program.

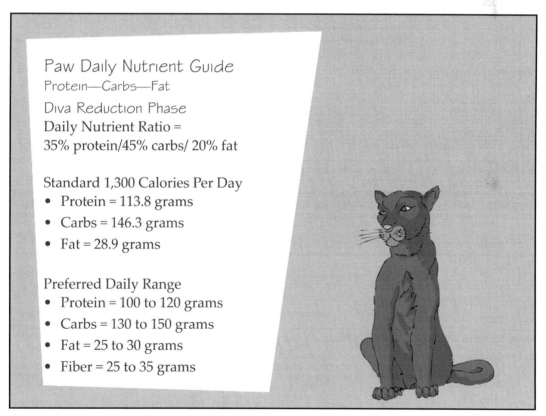

Paw Daily Nutrient Guide
Protein—Carbs—Fat

Diva Reduction Phase
Daily Nutrient Ratio =
35% protein/45% carbs/ 20% fat

Standard 1,300 Calories Per Day
- Protein = 113.8 grams
- Carbs = 146.3 grams
- Fat = 28.9 grams

Preferred Daily Range
- Protein = 100 to 120 grams
- Carbs = 130 to 150 grams
- Fat = 25 to 30 grams
- Fiber = 25 to 35 grams

Daily nutrient ratio: protein/carbohydrates/fat
- As stated in the beginning of this section, your nutrient ratio will be 35% protein/45% carbohydrates/20% fat.

- The Menu Plan for Fat Loss (PART FIVE) provides you with reduction meal options and recipes (pages 167-205), with complete instructions and guides based on the MY DIVA DIET regimen of four to five small meals per day.
  - The daily menu plan is broken down into four meal groups, each with twelve options, to give you a variety of choices for each of your four daily meals. We also provide target calories and nutrient breakdowns for each meal group so that you will stay within your daily total nutrient ratio range:
    - Breakfast = **323** calories: 20 grams protein; 45 grams carbs; 7 grams fat
    - Lunch = **343** calories: 35 grams protein; 35 grams carbs; 7 grams fat
    - Snack = **254** calories: 15 grams protein; 35 grams carbs; 6 grams fat
    - Supper = **370** calories: 40 grams protein; 25 grams carbs; 10 grams fat
- You can interchange some meals as long as you end up with the proper daily calories, ratio, and number of meals. If you keep within each meal calorie total and ratio breakdown, you will be fine (who said you can only have eggs or oatmeal for breakfast?). The only rule is that you limit your carbohydrate intake in the evening.
- You can also interchange some meals for a pure protein shake, smoothie, or green drink. This is good for when you don't have time for a full meal or are not that hungry.

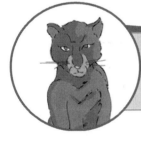

If you remember to have eggs, fish or lean poultry in 2 of your 4 meals, you will get the proper amount of protein each day. Dairy and plant foods have lower amounts, but they do add up.

Number of meals per day
- Eat frequent small meals throughout the day, including snacks.
- Four meals per day every three to four hours is best and will ensure that you keep a steady blood glucose level, which helps with fat loss and energy.

Meal timing
- Meal timing is up to you. Everyone's schedule is different. Just remember to eat every three to four hours.

When creating your own reduction meal plans, use the Diva Reduction Pyramid (p. 31 & 166).

36

- It's okay to add a snack as a fifth meal just in case you could not consume your total calories, or if you are hungry.
- Try to eat larger meals in the morning or afternoon. Reserve dinner for a nice piece of lean protein and some great-tasting fresh vegetables.

Meal size (portion control)
- Eating frequent small meals will also help you avoid overeating at any given meal. If you are tempted to eat too much at one time, just remember that you can eat again in three hours!

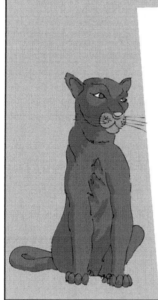

Paw Portion Guide

- Protein (fish, poultry, beef) should consist of no more than 3 to 5 oz. per meal.
- Eggs should be 5 whites or 2 whole eggs.
- Plant protein portions should be 1/2 cup for legumes and about 1 to 2 oz. for nuts and seeds.
- Carbs like rice, oats, and other whole grains should be no more than 1 cup.
- Fruit and veggies are great in all amounts and colors— the more fruit and veggies, the better.
- Fat will fall into place (added fat—like olive oil, salad dressing, and others should be no more than 2 Tbsp. at a time).

Factor #3: Quality and Purity of Calories

You should always monitor the quality and purity of your calories. This is crucial—not only for fat loss, but more importantly for health—"you are what you eat!"

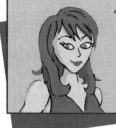

"Take the plunge and choose foods in their natural states that are fresh, organic, and kosher. You will not only reap the rewards of better health & fitness, but you will also help our environment and discourage mass production of animals for food (and reduce cruelty to animals)!"

Junk food (fast food, pizza, ice cream, potato chips, cookies, candy, donuts, etc.)
- Junk food is out—you may have it in the Diva Maintenance Phase, but only rarely.
- Desserts should be avoided for all of Phase One.
- Fruit or yogurt can be used for sweet-tooth cravings. If that is not enough, then use the Diva Smart Diet Cheat Sheet in PART FIVE (pages 216-219) for some good ideas on cheating.

Total daily fat intake (grams)
- Total daily fat grams should be limited to no more than 30 grams per day in Phase One (even the good fats—like olive oil, omega-3's, omega-6's, safflower, soybean, and sunflower oil—which we never want you to eliminate from your diet).
- In Phase Two you can have more fat grams per day, but they should be good fats and you need to control the quantity.

Total daily sugar intake (grams)
- You get plenty of sugar in foods naturally, so any added sugar should be kept to a bare minimum (50 grams per day or less).
- In the Diva Reduction Phase, only four extra sweetener products are allowed for now. You can use honey, agave nectar, natural fruit spreads, and applesauce, but keep them to a minimum. In Phase Two you can also use these and occasionally use other products containing sugar—be aware of the high caloric content and other problems associated with sugar.
- Avoid table sugar and products containing sugar and sugar derivatives.
- Sugar will always be a concern, especially if you consume packaged products. If you stay clear of most man-made food products you can assume that your sugar intake will be low unless you add table sugar to your tea, coffee, or cereal, or you consume syrup, molasses, jam, or similar products.
- After you remove sugar from your diet you will lose weight faster and feel much better, and with time you may no longer crave sugar.

Sugar substitutes intake (artificial sweeteners)
- MY DIVA DIET advises against using sugar substitutes in Phase One and Phase Two.
- Watch for sugar substitutes in packaged foods and drinks—they are everywhere.

Total daily sodium intake (milligrams)
- Sodium intake should be close to 1 milligram per calorie consumed (or less). If you eat real foods and stay away from (or are extremely selective in choosing) packaged foods, then your sodium level should be acceptable in both phases.
  - Sodium and sodium derivatives (which can be harmful) are found in many packaged, processed, and man-made food products.
- Another way to keep your sodium in check is to be selective in your use of seasonings, dips, dressings, sauces, and condiments. If you need that salty flavor, use sea salt or kosher salt in small amounts.

Quality protein intake
- Keep your meats to lean, non-processed choices like chicken and turkey (skinless white meat).
- Beef should be consumed only once per month or less.
- Limit whole eggs because of their high fat and cholesterol. You can have egg whites—they are a great source of protein without any fat or cholesterol.
- No pork.
- Avoid meat products. Occasional quality lunch meat (like Boar's Head or fresh deli meats) may be used, but stick with chicken or turkey breast.
- Stay away from processed fish, canned meats, bologna, ham, pastrami, and roast beef.
- No sausage, bacon, hot dogs, or veggie dogs for now.
- Jerky or smoked salmon—not yet (in Phase Two you can be more lax, but remain cautious).
- Plant protein (legumes, nuts, and seeds) is always an excellent choice for protein, fiber, and many other nutrients as long as its sources are natural and fresh.
  - Monitor the companies that sell you these foods.
  - Legumes should be fresh. If canned, check the ingredients.
  - Peas should be fresh but frozen is okay if the ingredients are few and pure.
  - Nuts and seeds are best when organic and raw. Make sure nut butters are pure (only one or two ingredients).
- Plant protein products allowed in the Diva Reduction Phase include only seven for now: soy milk, soy yogurt, soy butter, soy cheese, tofu, hummus, and nut butters. Just ensure their quality, as they must be pure and clean—check the ingredients!

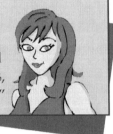

"How could any diet program not allow you to eat potatoes? When baked or boiled they are fat free and full of potassium, vitamins C and B6, and fiber, as well as other nutrients."

Quality carbohydrate intake

- Whole grains (not refined grains) are very nutritious—they are good for you and are not fattening, as some would have you believe. Just keep your portions from one-half to one cup at a time during Phase One (later you can have more).
  - Even though most white rice is processed, it is acceptable occasionally. Brown and wild rice are healthier choices.
  - Stay clear of wheat for now and choose gluten-free products.
- Fresh vegetables and fruits are always great—you can never go wrong choosing a variety (including watermelon, bananas, potatoes, and carrots).
- Dried fruit is fine in moderation, but it is high in calories and in Phase One includes only four: figs, raisins, dates, and prunes.
- Be sure to avoid dried fruit with added trans fats, sugars, and other impure ingredients.

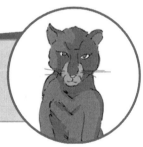

When choosing fruits and vegetables, go for colors—red, orange, yellow, green, blue/purple, and even white. Each color is a pigment that signifies the presence of certain antioxidants, vitamins, and minerals.

Quality fat intake

- Keep good fats up. But remember that in the Diva Reduction Phase you must limit them to 30 grams per day.
- Keep bad fats down.
  - Stay away from trans fats and hydrogenated oils.
  - Avoid foods that contain high amounts of saturated fats and cholesterol.

- Avoid bacon, sausage, and processed meats.
- Limit fatty cuts of beef, poultry with skin, egg yolks, butter, cream, cheese, and whole milk.
- Be selective when adding oils, nuts, butters, and sauces to your meals.

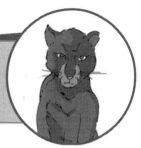

See Diva Reduction Good Food Choices At-a-Glance—PART SIX (pgs. 229-253) for more details on quality protein, carbohydrates, and fats.

Total daily dairy intake
- Dairy and dairy products for the Diva Reduction Phase include only eleven for now (and no more than one to two small portions per day): low-fat milk, low-fat cottage cheese, low-fat plain yogurt, low-fat cream cheese, low-fat sour cream, real butter, skim cheese, string cheese, and Parmesan, Romano, and feta cheese (other cheese can be added later).
  - Keep in mind that with a couple of slices of regular cheese you can end up consuming 18 grams of fat, 14 grams of protein, and 340 milligrams of sodium. And, some cheese includes other ingredients that you shouldn't eat at all.
- You should choose non-fat dairy and dairy products. This will lower your fat intake a few grams per day.
- Cow's milk and milk products are not the only sources of dairy—sheep and goat products are an optional source.
- You can substitute soy milk or soy products and rice milk for any dairy product.

Clean and pure calories
- In the Diva Reduction Phase you will be strict. Choose natural over processed foods, fresh over dead, organic over non-organic, kosher over non-kosher.
- You should limit your consumption of packaged, frozen, and canned foods.
  - The exceptions to the canned-food rule are canned legumes (plain of course), canned tuna in water, and some healthy canned soups.
  - Cheat times are the other exception.

41

- There are also quite a few frozen foods that are okay, including peas, corn, and fruits. However, the only ingredient in these products should be the food itself.
- If you do choose packaged foods, look for five ingredients or fewer and be wary of harmful additives, preservatives, and other ingredients commonly used in packaged foods and food products.

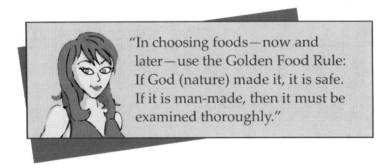

"In choosing foods—now and later—use the Golden Food Rule: If God (nature) made it, it is safe. If it is man-made, then it must be examined thoroughly."

White flour intake (bread, cereal, crackers, noodles, pasta, pastries, tortillas, etc.)
- MY DIVA DIET is a flourless diet plan for Phase One. White flour is out for now and so are other flours, even if they are made with healthy foods like wheat, rice, corn (masa), spelt, rye, potatoes, or nuts (these can be added later).
- White flour may be used as a cheat in Phase Two, but it will never be a big part of your diet again.
- No breads of any kind in Phase One—Diva Reduction (you will be able to add them later, but even then you should choose whole grain, high protein, and high fiber).
- Avoid flour products like pancakes, waffles, muffins, tortillas, etc. in Phase One.
- In Phase One you will be able to have grain products, but only whole grain and sprouted (baked—never fried—where applicable), and only seven for now: rice milk, rice cakes, corn thins, spelt cakes, sprouted corn tortillas, mochi, and some cereals (see the Diva Reduction Safe Cereals List—PART SIX, pages 254-255).
- It's best for now to limit cereals to oatmeal, quinoa and quinoa flakes, cream of rice and cream of buckwheat, and Nu-World Foods Amaranth Berry Delicious and Erewhon Organic Crispy Brown Rice (unless you can find others that meet the MY DIVA DIET Food Criteria—Diva Reduction Pyramid, pages 31 & 166).

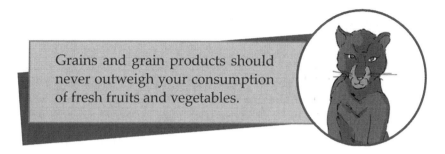

Grains and grain products should never outweigh your consumption of fresh fruits and vegetables.

Total daily fiber intake (grams)
- Fiber will always be a priority for initial and long-term fat loss and health. Try to consume 25 to 35 grams per day.
- The MY DIVA DIET slogan for Phase One and Phase Two is "Fiber, fiber, and more fiber!"

Food, sports, energy, and protein bars
- Stay away from these in Phase One. Most are just glorified candy bars anyway.
- In Phase Two you can use food, sports, energy, and protein bars in an emergency situation, like when you are forced to eat on the run. They can be used as substitutes for any meal—just ensure the quality of the ingredients used.

Sauces, salad dressing, dips, and condiment intake
- In Phase One you will be limited to some salad dressings, special mayonnaise, salsa, mustard, horseradish, and marinara sauce. You may have others if you have examined their ingredients—just use small amounts.
- In Phase Two you can add more as long as their ingredients are pure. Be aware that most have a high fat and sugar content, and look for any preservatives, fillers, and other unfamiliar ingredients.

Cooking and seasoning (fruits, vegetables, herbs, spices)
- Always monitor how your food is prepared, whether you are eating at home or in a restaurant. This is a major key to MY DIVA DIET success.
- Ask questions when you dine out—it is your body and your money. You don't want eating out to interfere with your progress.
- Refer to PART FIVE (pages 206-215) for more on food preparation and for dining out see PART SIX (pages 268-276).

Supplement intake (vitamins, minerals, and others)
- Vitamins, minerals, and other supplements may be necessary, especially in the Diva Reduction Phase, when you have reduced your calorie intake and perhaps also your nutrient intake. On the other hand, you are eating foods that have more nutritional value, so you may actually be getting more nutrients than before.
- You are eating quality foods, so don't overdose on supplements. A good multivitamin and some extra water-soluble vitamins are good.
  - Keep in mind that not all vitamins are made the same—some are natural and some synthetic. Always choose natural supplements.

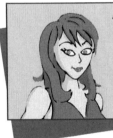

"There is no quick-fix to fat loss or vibrant health. Stay away from any pill that is marketed that way, especially diet pills. Be careful of so-called amino acids and other herbs on the market today. There are too many to list—we want you to be aware."

Factor #4: Restrictive and Unbalanced Dieting

- Stay away from starvation plans—or any diet that limits good foods. They don't work and they put you at risk for health issues and/or yo-yo dieting.
- Stay away from fad diets, gimmicks, and false promises for the same reason.
- Stay away from pills and potions for fat loss—these can be dangerous.

Factor #5: Exercise

- Get moving—the fat will come off faster and you'll look and feel better.
- Try to add an effective and efficient exercise program to your weekly schedule.
- Hire a fitness professional to help you get on the right track. This will ensure that you don't waste time or money and will help you avoid injury and imbalance.

Maybe you've only been on the program for two weeks and you are thinking: "This isn't working." That is normal in our society—most of us are impatient and want instant gratification. But just remember how long it took for you to get out of shape in the first place. Two weeks is not sufficient for any proper diet program to take effect.

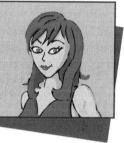

"If you don't reach your weight-loss goals as quickly as you'd like, don't be tempted to fall back into old habits. If you fall off the 'diet wagon' at any time, dust yourself off and get back on!"

The best way to lose weight is to do it slowly, for two main reasons:
- It is safer and healthier, and the weight loss will most definitely be fat.
- You're creating a new lifestyle for yourself—the changes you make are long-term habits with diet and exercise which will help you get healthy & fit—for life!

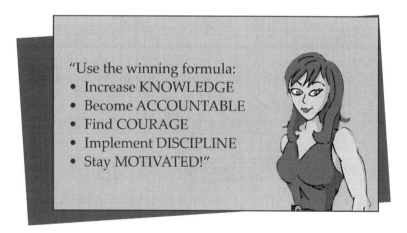

"Use the winning formula:
- Increase KNOWLEDGE
- Become ACCOUNTABLE
- Find COURAGE
- Implement DISCIPLINE
- Stay MOTIVATED!"

Phase Two: Diva Maintenance Pyramid
(MY DIVA DIET Food Criteria)

1,400 to 1,600 Calories Per Day (Average)
- 20 to 35% protein/45 to 65% carbs/20 to 30% fat
- 4 to 5 meals per day
- Clean and pure foods
- Natural, fresh, organic, and kosher foods

- High in water intake
- High in nutrients
- High in antioxidants
- High in real/live pure organic foods
- High in alkaline-forming foods (low acidic-forming)
- High in the proper balance of protein, carbs, and fat
- High in fiber

- Alcohol-free (may add in moderation)
- Low in all types of flour and flour products/white flour-free
- Partially gluten-free (may add whole wheat now)
- Free of artificial ingredients
- Free of genetically modified foods
- Junk food-free

- Extra low in processed and refined foods
- Low in food additives and preservatives
- Naturally low-glycemic

- Low dairy
- Low sugar
- Low sodium
- Low in saturated fats and cholesterol

Phase Two: Diva Maintenance—For Life

The second phase of the MY DIVA DIET program is Phase Two—Diva Maintenance. This phase is to make sure you preserves what you have accomplished in the Diva Reduction Phase. You'll go on doing what you know is right, but you'll also have more leeway to deviate from the strict plan of Phase One.

Maintenance is a lifestyle. We can help you with more information (and menu plans that go beyond PART FIVE) via our website at www.MyDivaDiet.com.

In Phase Two—Diva Maintenance you can eat more—about 1,400 to 1,600 calories per day, depending on your activity level (for women who are very active, daily calories may increase as high as 2,000 per day).

Some of you may be more comfortable staying at 1,200 to 1,300 calories per day (as in the Diva Reduction Phase). That's fine, but never go lower than that. Usually what happens anyway is that one day we may consume 1,200 calories and the next 1,600, and then the following day 1,300. That is why it's always best to work within a range of calories and not get locked into a single number.

During the Diva Maintenance Phase, assuming 1,600 calories per day, if you divide your daily calories by four, you should consume about 400 calories per meal. The approximate targeted nutrient ratio is:
* 20 to 35% protein/45 to 65% carbohydrates/20 to 30% fat (these may vary and fluctuate)

In Phase Two—Diva Maintenance you can also cheat more, making selections from the Diva Smart Diet Cheat Sheet—PART FIVE (pages 216-219) or by creating your own cheating options, or even once in a while—one to two times per month—deviating from the program.

The following Paw Cheat Guide gives you some examples of ways you can relax the rules occasionally in Phase Two—Diva Maintenance.

Paw Diet Cheat Guide for Phase Two—
Diva Maintenance ✱

#1   You have a high-fat cappuccino or non-fresh juice.

#2   You eat a little too much—or not enough—one day.

#3   Your nutrient ratio is not on track—too many carbs.

#4   Maybe you have only 2 to 3 meals one day.

#5   You skip breakfast or eat a large dinner.

#6   Maybe you have a large portion one day.

#7   You are tempted by junk food as a cheat.

#8   You don't ensure the quality of your foods, eating non-organic, or using white flour instead of whole grain.

#9   Maybe you choose a fatty sauce, salad dressing, or dip.

#10 You eat at a restaurant and are not selective.

#11 You have too many cocktails.

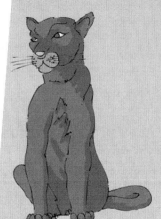

––––––––––

✱ Try to cheat in healthier ways and only 1 to 2 times per month.

The Five Factors in the Diva Maintenance Phase

(Per the Diva 32-Question Diet Quiz—PART THREE, pages 61 to 83)

Factor #1: Liquid Consumption

- Plenty of water—forever!
- Liquid intake should be the same as in Phase One. An occasional deviation may be okay from time to time—just don't get into the habit of choosing poor-quality liquids.
- Alcohol in moderation is okay—create boundaries!

Factor #2: Quantity and Distribution of Calories

Daily caloric intake (overeating or undereating)
- In Phase One you kept your daily calories low and controlled for fat reduction. In Phase Two you can increase your caloric intake to 1,400 to 1,600 calories per day, depending on your activity level, goals, medical condition, etc.
- By this time you should know quite a bit about foods and their makeup (calories, protein, carbohydrates, fat, fiber, etc.). You will be a walking food dictionary! You will be able to look at a plate and accurately estimate calories and nutrient grams. If you have not reached this level yet—hang in there—you will soon!
- Knowledge is power, so remain in a learning mode: keep gathering information about foods and nutrition.

Daily nutrient ratio: protein/carbohydrates/fat
- Your daily nutrient ratio was strict in Phase One—Diva Reduction, but you will have more flexibility in Phase Two—Diva Maintenance. Follow this guide:

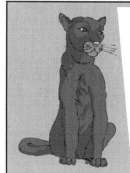

Paw Nutrient Ratio Guide

Diva Reduction Phase:
35% protein/45% carbs/20% fat (or close)
Diva Maintenance Phase:
20 to 35% protein/45 to 65% carbs/20 to 30% fat *
    * Maintenance ratio can fluctuate
    * Extra-lean Divas can go as low as 15% fat

- You will always consume protein, carbohydrates, and fats—and always in the proper ratio. And since you have been eating so many fruits and vegetables in Phase One, you will crave them now.
- As far as a menu plan in the Diva Maintenance Phase, you can use the Diva Reduction Meal Options and Recipes in PART FIVE (pages 167-205) and make some adjustments.
- You can continue to interchange meal options and use protein shakes, smoothies, or green drinks as a meal replacement. It's better to eat than starve.
- In Phase Two you can now have starchy carbohydrates at dinner, like bread, pasta, potatoes, and rice—just don't go crazy!

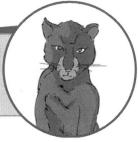

When creating your own daily menu plans for maintenance, use the Diva Maintenance Pyramid (PART TWO, p. 46).

Number of meals per day
- Continue eating about four small meals throughout the day.
- You can add one or two (healthy) snacks.

Meal timing
- Meal timing and eating frequent small meals throughout the day should always be part of your life. By now you should be hungry every three to four hours.
- Continue to consume your larger meals in the morning or afternoon. At dinner, continue eating a lean piece of protein and fresh vegetables.
- Once in a while, a big dinner is fine in Phase Two.

Meal size (portion control)
- You will always follow guidelines for portion control—to maintain what you've worked for and to keep from overeating—and now you know how to do that well. Use the same rules as in the Diva Reduction Phase, but you can have a little more food in the Diva Maintenance Phase.
- By this time you should be used to smaller portions—and feel uncomfortable when you eat too much!

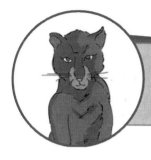

Continue to use the Paw Portion Guide from Phase One (p. 37) and a more thorough one can be found in PART FOUR (p. 104-107).

Factor #3: Quality and Purity of Calories

Junk food (fast food, pizza, ice cream, potato chips, cookies, candy, donuts, etc.)
• Junk food is still not recommended. However, if you must have some, make sure it is on special occasions (once per month or less) and be selective.
• Most desserts are really junk food, so continue to use the advice from Phase One and refer to the Diva Smart Diet Cheat Sheet, being selective (by now you should also have created your own smart diet cheating list to give you more variety when "you feel the need to be bad").

Total daily fat intake (grams)
• In Phase One you counted fat grams (even the good ones) and kept them at 30 grams or less. You also kept most of your fat intake to good quality. In Phase Two you have a little more flexibility on total fat grams per day. Just don't go overboard and you won't gain the fat back—try to keep your fat grams close to 30 grams per day most of the time.

Total daily sugar intake (grams)
• By now sugar is not a big part of your diet. Since you get plenty of sweet from foods naturally and you enjoy the taste of foods without added sugars, continue to stay away from table sugar and products that contain sugar and sugar derivatives.
• Extra sweetener products for Phase One included only four: honey, agave nectar, natural fruit spreads, and applesauce. In Phase Two it is still a good idea to keep to this rule. You can also use other products that are natural and low in sugar—read the labels.
• Fresh fruit is always good when you want something sweet.

Sugar substitutes intake (artificial sweeteners)
- Continue to stay away from artificially made sweeteners and be leery of those claiming to be made of natural ingredients. This includes those on the market today and any future products that may come along.

Total daily sodium intake (milligrams)
- In Phase One you monitored your daily sodium intake and kept it to around 1,300 milligrams (depending on your daily caloric intake). Continue this pattern—you probably noticed that a lot of bloating went away by eating pure and clean foods. Better yet, by now you really taste your food—not what is put on it (broccoli and fresh fish are delicious, rice and potatoes have their own special flavor).
- By Phase Two you have also turned the corner in the way you season your foods: you use fruits, vegetables, herbs, and spices.
- You've learned to actively dislike the taste of processed, packaged, and man-made foods, which are full of sodium, sodium derivatives (most of which are not good), fat and sugar. Keep it up—there's no turning back!

Quality protein intake
- Continue to keep your meats to lean, non-processed poultry (including occasional skinless dark meat now), and fresh fish.
- Beef should still be eaten only once per month or less. Beef is good but it should be considered a luxury item, not part of your daily menu. Save it for special occasions and enjoy it.
- Whole eggs can be consumed a little more often now.
- Pork is still not recommended.
- Meat products for Phase One included only one: quality chicken or turkey breast lunch meat like Boar's Head or fresh deli types. In Phase Two you can now add good-quality deli roast beef occasionally.
- Continue to stay away from canned meats, bologna, ham, and pastrami.
- Continue to avoid regular sausage or bacon.
- Kosher hot dogs and veggie dogs are all right once in a while.
- Occasional turkey sausage is okay if the ingredients are pure.
- Occasional organic turkey jerky is acceptable, as well as smoked salmon.

- Continue to keep in mind the high sodium in all meat products, including the ones we are listing as acceptable once in a while: lunch meat, kosher hot dogs, turkey sausage, turkey jerky, and smoked salmon.
- Make sure you select meat products with pure ingredients.
- Plant protein like legumes, nuts, and seeds should continue to be a part of your daily diet as they offer many nutrients, as well as fiber.
  - Keep in mind the high fat in nuts and seeds (even though it is good fat).
  - Continue to monitor the companies that sell you plant protein products.
- In Phase One we included seven plant protein products: soy milk, soy yogurt, soy butter, soy cheese, tofu, hummus, and nut butters. In Phase Two you can add more—just read the labels to ensure the ingredients are pure and that plant protein is the main ingredient.

Quality carbohydrate intake

- Whole grains and whole-grain products (rarely, if ever refined) should be a big part of your diet from now on.
  - In the Diva Reduction Phase we allowed white rice. This is still fine in moderation. Be selective when adding other refined grains to your diet.
  - You can now add whole wheat to your diet—but continue to choose gluten-free products most of the time.
  - Now that you know that grains are good for you and not fattening, continue to try a variety. They give you great energy and many important nutrients. Keep them at one to two cups at a time.
- Continue your high intake of all fruits and vegetables. By now you are enjoying their diversity of bright colors and delicious flavors and having fun experimenting with new varieties—while adding essential nutrients to your diet.
- In Phase One dried fruit choices included only four: figs, raisins, dates, and prunes. In Phase Two more varieties of dried fruit are acceptable—just be sure that the ingredients are fruit only. This is a good way to get your snack without turning to junk food or sugary snack items.

> Remember that the colors (pigments) of fruits and vegetables—red, orange, yellow, green, blue/purple, and even white—indicate important nutritional components for your diet.

Quality fat intake
- You will always have fat in your diet, and by this time you will know which fats are good and which ones are bad. You will also be more aware of fat grams.
- In Phase Two you can have between 30 to 50 grams of fat per day. Just remain vigilant when deciding on foods with fat in them, or when adding fats to your meals.

> Continue to use the Diva Reduction Good Food Choices At-a-Glance—PART SIX (pgs. 229-253) to aid you in choosing the proper protein, carbs, and fats.

Total daily dairy intake
- In Phase One dairy products included only eleven (and only one to two small servings per day): low-fat milk, low-fat cottage cheese, low-fat plain yogurt, low-fat cream cheese, low-fat sour cream, real butter, skim cheese, string cheese, and Parmesan, Romano and feta cheese. This is plenty of dairy to choose from.
- In Phase Two you can add other types of cheese. Keep in mind that cheese is high in fat and sodium and some cheese has ingredients you shouldn't eat.
- As in Phase One, remember that dairy products from sheep and goats are also options.
- As in Phase One, you can always skip the dairy and substitute soy milk, soy products, and rice milk.

Clean and pure calories
- Continue to monitor the quality of your calories forever.
- In Phase One you have been strict, selecting natural, fresh, organic, and kosher foods, and learning that good foods taste great. You will have little desire to return to fake, unnatural, processed, and unfit foods.
- Continue to read labels to ensure the foods you eat are clean and pure of any harmful preservatives and additives.
- By eating clean and pure foods, you not only look better but also feel better about your health, your body, yourself, and your environment. Keep it up!

White flour intake (bread, cereals, crackers, noodles, pasta, pastries, tortillas, etc.)

- Breads can be added now, in moderation. If you are not gluten intolerant, you can add whole grain breads from wheat and other grains (sprouted breads are best).

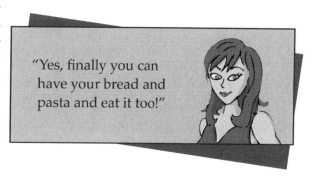

"Yes, finally you can have your bread and pasta and eat it too!"

  - Make sure you keep bread in its proper place—eat bread only a few times per week (and not the entire loaf). The rule here is "less is better."

- Be careful when allowing flour products back into your diet.
- White flour in Phase Two is still not a good idea, but occasionally (as a cheat) some exceptions are no-salt sourdough pretzels, white pasta, and sourdough bread.
- Grain products in Phase One included only seven: rice milk, rice cakes, corn thins, spelt cakes, sprouted corn tortillas, mochi, and some cereals. In Phase Two you should still watch your consumption of grain products, the majority of which should be made from whole grains, sprouted grains, and/or grains that are stone ground. But you can add other foods made with quality flours beyond white and wheat, like rice, corn (masa), spelt, rye, potatoes, nuts, etc. Again, they should be baked—never fried.
- For cereals, continue to use the Diva Reduction Safe Cereals List in PART SIX (pages 254-255). You can also add others if you have done your homework and select ones that fit the food criteria found in the Diva Reduction Pyramid or Diva Maintenance Pyramid (pages 31, 46, & 166).

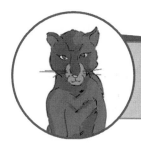

As in Phase One, continue to be careful that grains and grain products do not replace fresh fruits and vegetables as carbohydrate choices.

Total daily fiber intake (grams)
- Fiber will always be a priority for initial and long-term fat loss and health, and by now you will know which foods supply fiber.
- The MY DIVA DIET slogan continues to apply: "Fiber, fiber, fiber!"

Food, sports, energy, and protein bars
- You can use these in Phase Two. Just remember that they are not what they are advertised to be—they are not real foods. Put them in their proper place—as an emergency choice once in a while, and be selective.

Sauces, salad dressing, dips, and condiment intake
- It's best to stay with what you used in Phase One. But you have more flexibility now and you read labels like an expert! So once in a while you can deviate as long as you are aware of ingredients. Read labels!

Cooking and seasoning (fruits, vegetables, herbs, spices)
- You will always want to monitor how your food is prepared, whether you are eating at home or in a restaurant. By this time you understand what can "kill" a food and what can make it more alive and flavorful. Keep up your healthful cooking—and continue to take charge of your body. If you need help on food preparation and dining out see PART FIVE (pages 206-215) and PART SIX (pages 268-276).

Supplement intake (vitamins, minerals, and others)
- A good multi-vitamin and some extra water-soluble vitamins are good to take on a regular basis. Even if you are eating more in Phase Two, it is still difficult to get all the nutrients you need for optimal fitness and healthy levels. Just don't go crazy here—you can overdose on vitamins (especially the fat-soluble ones).
- Continue to choose natural over synthetic supplements every time.

Factor #4: Restrictive and Unbalanced Dieting
- You have now lost fat without starving, limiting good foods, or resorting to fad diets, false promises, pills, or other weight-loss gimmicks; and you've even become healthier along the way.
- Continue to avoid starvation diets and other diets that limit healthy foods.
- Continue to avoid new fad diets, gimmicks and false promises.
- Don't be tempted by new "miracle" diet pills and weight-loss programs.

Factor #5: Exercise

- If you still have not started an exercise program:

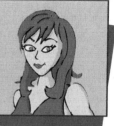

> "Hire a fitness professional who can guide and motivate you. This will be key in assuring that your fat loss and health goals are met and maintained."

- If you've implemented an exercise program and attained your goals:

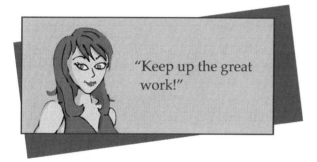

> "Keep up the great work!"

- And if you've reached your goals without exercise:

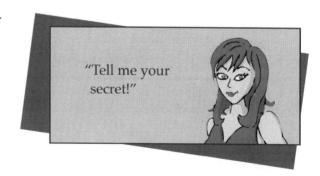

> "Tell me your secret!"

- Exercise should always be part of your life. If you've been exercising regularly for a while (more than three months), in Phase Two—Diva Maintenance you can back off a little and allow for breaks—like a week of recuperation, holidays, and special occasions.

Paw Diet Tools Guide

Look for our "diet tools," which can be used over and over to help you choose what to eat and aid you in creating your own Diva Meals and Diva Recipes, whether you are in the Phase Two—Diva Reduction or Phase Two—Diva Maintenance of the MY DIVA DIET program.

These tools include:

- Diva Reduction Pyramid and Diva Maintenance Pyramid—PART TWO (page 31 & 46 & 166)

- MY DIVA DIET Food Preparation, Cooking, and Meal Planning Guide—PART FIVE (pages 206-215)

- Diva Reduction Good Food Choices At-a-Glance— PART SIX (pages 229-253)

- Diva Reduction Safe Cereals List— PART SIX (pages 254-255)

- Diva Food Test and Paw Label Guide— PART SIX (pages 265-267)

- MY DIVA DIET Restaurant Eating Guide— PART SIX (pages 268-276)

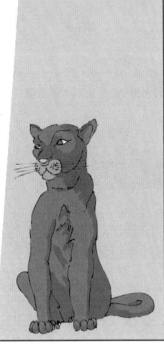

In the Diva Maintenance Phase you will have arrived at your body fat and health goals, or be well on your way. Congratulations!

You have created a new and healthy lifestyle with enough knowledge and discipline to continue doing all the right things, gaining more variety in the foods you eat, and knowing better than to fall for the latest dieting craze.

You are now convinced that there is no quick-fix to fat loss. But with Ms. Diva and Paw as your guides and your own hard work, you can be fit, healthy, and look awesome— so share this good news with your family and friends.

PART THREE

The Analysis

You never find yourself until you face the truth.

~ Pearl Bailey

MY DIVA DIET Analysis Overview

Every smart and successful woman who truly wants to improve significant personal areas of her life—the development of her character, relationships with others, her spiritual life—or who wants to see progress in more pragmatic areas—her career, financial planning, time management—will always begin with a thorough evaluation of her current condition. It is no different for women who want to transform their bodies into lean, healthy, sexy, more functional machines.

We start to become true Diva Dieters by changing our eating habits, and this type of change requires a complete and honest diet analysis.

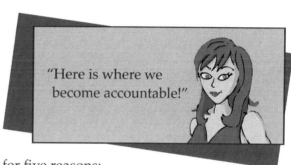

"Here is where we become accountable!"

A diet analysis is a very powerful tool for five reasons:

#1:   It gives you a true and precise picture of exactly what kinds of foods you're consuming (i.e. becoming aware of what you are putting into your body).

#2:   It will help you examine your overall eating and exercising practices.

#3:   It will reveal your strengths and weaknesses in specific areas of health & fitness.

#4:   It will ultimately help you create a new lifestyle incorporating proper eating and exercise.

#5:   It will serve as a tool to guide and keep you in line for the long term.

Think of your diet analysis as a map indicating "you are here." It will tell you where you are, how far you need to go, and how long your transformation process will take. This is the beginning of your success. After your analysis, you should seek accurate knowledge on how to change, and then you need to implement whatever changes are necessary. We know you have the courage to do so!

On the following pages the Diva 32-Question Diet Quiz will help you analyze your relationship to the Five Factors Affecting Body Fat and Health (PART ONE, pages 10-12). The Diva Diet Quiz will also introduce you to the Diet Villains (PART ONE, pages 15-19), some of which you may be battling today.

Follow these steps:
- Answer the 32 questions in the Diva Diet Quiz.
- Record your scores in the Diva Diet Quiz Scores section.
- Grade yourself in the Diva Diet Quiz Grades section (explanatory score summaries are provided.)
- Transfer your totals and other information to your workspace in PART EIGHT— Diva Worksheet #2 (pages 352-355). This will give you a quick glance at your results and help you note where you can make adjustments that will make a definite difference.

At this point you may decide that you have enough information for now—the quiz is very thorough and will give you insight into your eating and excercise patterns. Or you can take the information you've tracked and fix certain areas within the Five Factors to get results.

If you want a more precise picture of your total daily calorie and nutrient intake, you should do a three-day diet analysis to track actual calories and your nutrient ratio (see the 3-Day Diet Analysis and Food Diary Sheets in PART EIGHT—Diva Worksheet #3 and #4, pages 356-365).

You can always skip this section (PART THREE) and go directly to the Diva Reduction Meal Options and Diva Reduction Recipes (PART FIVE, pages 153-205) to get started, but his this is not recommended. Knowledge is power, and understanding your eating, and excercise habits will help you improve them now and in the future.

We at MY DIVA DIET advocate that you use this analysis not only when you begin the MY DIVA DIET program, but also periodically throughout the program to learn more about foods, add other foods to your daily diet, and—most importantly—stay on track.

Sometimes we get comfortable and end up gaining a few pounds back. If you do a quick analysis now and again, you may be amazed at how many calories (and what kind) have sneaked back in. You can also gauge other areas that affect *your* body fat and health.

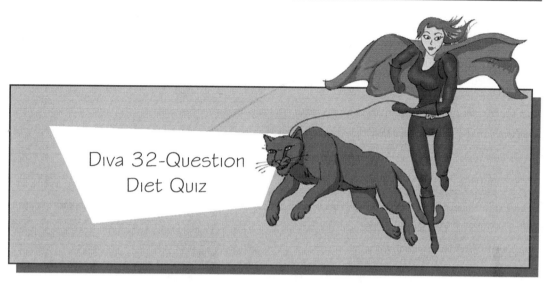

Instructions

There are 32 questions within the Five Factors Affecting Body Fat and Health in the Diva Diet Quiz.

- Make sure you answer every question.
- Answer each question honestly.
- Check only one answer for each question.
- Check the answer that best reflects your true eating and excercise habits—not according to a new diet plan, what you think you should eat, or what you plan on eating in the future.
- Under the Diva Diet Quiz Scores, record your scores and add them up (you will subtract a 35-point correction factor).
- Under the Diva Diet Quiz Grades, check your total to see how you did.
- Transfer your Diva Diet Quiz data to "MY Workspace" found in PART EIGHT to collect all your data in you very own personal health & fitness section.

Your Diva Diet Quiz Scores will help guide you into the right adjustments to reach your overall goal to getting fit the healthy, safe, and lasting way. Most questions are worth between +30 and -30 points. A few indicate more significant aspects of your diet (water and alcohol intake, clean and pure calories, fiber intake, restrictive and unbalanced dieting), so they are worth +50 to -50. Exercise ranges from +65 to –65, depending on the regularity of your habit.

In PART FOUR (pages 87-149) you will be able to explore each of the Diva Diet Quiz's 32 questions further. We have included the following:

- Notes explain why a particular question was important in your overall picture of dieting and health and provide you with other material relevant to that sub-topic.
- Rules give you guides to follow in each specific area.
- FYI's provide extra information to help you succeed.

"A fun thing would be to take the Diva Diet Quiz with some friends and compare your scores and which Diet Villains you most relate to."

Diva Diet Quiz

Factor #1: Liquid Consumption

1. Water

❑ I drink plenty of water—at least 8 to 10 cups per day = +50
❑ I drink water frequently = +20
❑ I drink water once in a while = 0
❑ I drink water only when I'm thirsty = -20
❑ I use water only in my coffee = -30
❑ I don't drink water—only other liquids = -35
❑ I use water only when I take a bath = -40
❑ I'm dehydrated all the time, like Pops = -50

Total #1 = _____

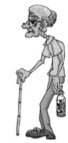

POPS

2. Coffee and other caffeinated drinks

❑ I don't drink coffee = 0
❑ I drink decaffeinated coffee = 0
❑ I drink coffee only on occasion = 0
❑ I drink coffee daily, but only 2 cups or less = 0
❑ I drink a lot of coffee daily (plain) = -5
❑ I drink coffee daily (with cream and/or sugar) = -15
❑ I drink mocha frappuccinos or other
high-calorie coffee drinks all the time = -20
❑ I drink many caffeinated energy drinks
and Caff is my hero = -20

Total #2 = _____

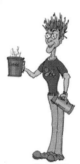

CAFF

3. Tea

❑ I drink herbal, green, black, and red tea = +20
❑ I drink green, black, and red tea = +15
❑ I drink only herbal tea = +10
❑ I don't drink tea = 0
❑ I drink tea with my sugar = -15

Total #3 = _____

4. Soda
   ❑ I don't drink soda at all   = +10
   ❑ I drink sodas only once in a while   = -5
   ❑ I drink only diet sodas   = -15
   ❑ I drink regular sodas quite often   = -15
   ❑ Like Pops, I choose soda as my favorite drink   = -20
                                              Total #4 = _____

5. Other drinks (sports drinks, powdered soft drinks, juice boxes, and other sugary drinks)
   ❑ I don't drink these at all   = +10
   ❑ I drink these only once in a while   = -5
   ❑ I drink other drinks like store-bought lemonade, orange drinks,
     grape juice, etc. (none of which are freshly squeezed)   = -10
   ❑ I drink these kinds of drinks but only those made
     with artificial sweeteners   = -10
                                              Total #5 = _____

6. Juice (fruit and vegetable): fresh vs. concentrated
   ❑ I have a juicer and drink only fresh-squeezed fruit and vegetable juices   = +15
   ❑ I drink only store-bought fresh fruit and vegetable juices   = +5
   ❑ I don't drink any juice at all (I'm kind of scared of that vegetable juice stuff) = 0
   ❑ I drink store-bought fruit and vegetable juices (not fresh) on occasion   = -5
   ❑ I drink fruit and vegetable juices in any form (vegetable, cranberry, apple,
     orange)—if it says "juice" I assume it is good for me   = -15
                                              Total #6 = _____

7. Meal replacement drinks (protein shakes, smoothies, and green drinks)
   ❑ I prefer to make my protein shakes, smoothies, and veggie drinks at home using
     only high-quality protein powder, water, fresh juice, and/or low-fat milk and
     yogurt or soy products, and fresh fruit and vegetables   = +15

❑ I drink other meal replacement drinks that are
    high in nutrients and low in sugar   = +10

❑ I drink liquid drinks that are low dairy, low sugar, and low fat
    (and most are full of nutrients and fiber)   = +10

❑ I don't drink protein shakes, smoothies, or green drinks at all   = 0

❑ I drink liquid meal drinks like Slim-Fast, Weight Watchers, etc.,
    but only once in a while   = -5

❑ I drink a lot of liquid meal drinks in any form   = -10

Total #7 = _____

8. Alcohol

❑ I don't drink alcohol at all   = +50

❑ I only drink alcohol on special occasions   = +20

❑ I drink alcohol rarely   = +10

❑ I drink wine once in a while   = 0

❑ I drink only wine and only a few times per week = -10

❑ I drink alcohol once a week (all kinds)   = -15

❑ I drink wine a lot   = -20

❑ I drink alcohol 2 to 3 times per week (a lot and all kinds) = -30

❑ I drink alcohol every day (a lot and all kinds) and would
    like to party with Al and Cole   = -50

Total #8 = _____

AL AND COLE

Factor #2: Quantity and Distribution of
                 Daily Calories

9. Daily caloric intake (overeating or
    undereating)

❑ I eat approximately 1,200 to 2,000 calories per day = +20

❑ I don't know how many calories per day I eat
    (but I do eat)   +10

❑ I don't know how many calories per day I eat
    (and I hardly eat)   = -10

❑ I overeat (more than 3,000 calories per day). I
    have no control, just like Joe Stufft   = -30

JOE STUFFT

❑ I undereat (less than 1,000 calories per day).
  I starve myself, and Girlie Die is my role model   = -30
                              Total #9 = _____

**GIRLIE DIE AND
HER POODLE, IT**

10. Daily nutrient ratio: (35% protein/45% carbs/20% fat)
  ❑ I eat a balanced diet from all these nutrients and at this ratio
    (or close to this ratio)   = +30
  ❑ I eat a balanced diet from all these nutrients
    but am unsure about the ratio   = +20
  ❑ I don't pay attention to what I eat   = 0
  ❑ I don't know the difference between protein, carbs, or fat   = -10
  ❑ I have no clue what this question is about   = -20
  ❑ I am currently on a high-protein, high-fat, no-carb diet   = -30
                              Total #10 = _____

11. Number of meals per day (including snacks)
  ✳ If you eat 3 or more meals per day, fill in the following:
  ❑ I eat ____ meals per day
    ✳ Give yourself 5 points for each meal   = +__
  ✳ If you eat fewer than 3 meals per day, choose from the following:
  ❑ I eat 2 meals per day   = -10
  ❑ I eat only 1 meal per day   = -20
                              Total #11 = _____

12. Meal timing
  ✳ When do you eat the most?
  ❑ Breakfast   = +15
  ❑ Lunch   = +15
  ❑ Snacks   = +5
  ❑ Dinner   = -10
  ❑ Late night   = -15
                              Total #12 = _____

13. Meal size (portion control)

* When do you stop eating at a given meal?

- ❑ I never eat until I feel too full   = +20
- ❑ I rarely eat until I feel too full   = +10
- ❑ I don't pay attention—I just eat   = -5
- ❑ I sometimes eat until I feel too full   = -10
- ❑ I eat every morsel on my plate, no matter what   = -10
- ❑ What is portion control?   = -20
- ❑ I eat until I feel too full all the time   = -30

Total #13 = _____

Factor #3: Quality and Purity of Calories

14. Junk food (fast food, pizza, ice cream, potato chips, cookies, candy, donuts, etc.)

- ❑ I never eat junk food   = +30
- ❑ I rarely eat junk food   = +15
- ❑ I eat junk food only on special occasions or under certain circumstances   = +5
- ❑ I eat junk food once per month or less   = 0
- ❑ I eat junk food once per week   = -10
- ❑ I eat junk food a few times per week   = -20
- ❑ I eat junk food every day   = -25
- ❑ I love junk food—it's my main choice of food. As Junkster says, "Junk food rules"   = -30

JUNKSTER

Total #14 = _____

15. Total daily fat intake (grams)

- ❑ I eat around 30 grams of fat per day   = +15
- ❑ I eat low fat   = +5
- ❑ I have no clue how many fat grams I eat per day   = -10
- ❑ I eat a lot fat each day (over 50 grams)   = -15

Total #15 = _____

16. Total daily sugar intake (grams)

- ❏ I eat less than 50 grams of sugar each day   = +30
- ❏ I rarely eat sugar or any sugary kinds of products
  or packaged foods   = +20
- ❏ I eat low sugar (hardly any fat-free high-sugar products,
  very few packaged foods, no table sugar, syrup, jams, etc.)
       = +10
- ❏ I eat sugar and products made with sugar once in a while   = -10
- ❏ I have no clue how much sugar I consume each day   = -20
- ❏ I consume a lot of sugar and sugar-type products each day.
  I want Shoog's candy bar and soda right now!   = -30

Total #16 = _____

SHOOG

17. Sugar substitutes (artificial sweeteners)

- ❏ I never use artificial sweeteners or products made with them   = +15
- ❏ I really don't know   = -5
- ❏ I use these only once in a while   = -10
- ❏ I use these and consume products made with these quite often   = -15

Total #17= _____

18. Total daily sodium intake (milligrams)

- ❏ I eat less than 1,600 mg of sodium each day (most of it from natural foods)
  and/or I occasionally use kosher or sea salt   = +15
- ❏ I eat low sodium (I don't salt my food, I rarely eat at restaurants, and I don't eat
  processed, canned, or frozen foods and very few sauces, creams, etc.)   = +10
- ❏ I use salt only to shake over my shoulder for luck   = 0
- ❏ I have no clue how much sodium I consume each day = -10
- ❏ I do use salt in my cooking and sometimes salt my food,
  but I don't eat a lot of processed foods   = -10
- ❏ I cook with a lot of salt and eat a lot of processed,
  canned, and frozen foods   = -15
- ❏ I eat high sodium—I love salt and put
  it on everything, just like Sodi Sumo   = -15

Total #18 = _____   **SODI SUMO**

19. Quality protein intake
- ❏ I eat lean protein, like chicken and turkey breast, and occasionally lean cuts of beef. I eat lean fresh fish. I prefer egg whites to whole eggs. And I eat plenty of legumes, peas, nuts, and seeds as my main protein choices   = +30
- ❏ I eat good and bad protein choices   = +10
- ❏ I eat only dark poultry meat with the skin, burgers, shellfish, and whole eggs. What are legumes? I eat roasted salted nuts, and I use seeds only in my garden   = -30

Total #19 = _____

20. Quality carbohydrate intake
- ❏ I eat only whole grains (like oats, rice, corn, etc.) and only whole-grain products like whole-wheat breads, spinach pasta, etc.), as well as a variety of plain fresh fruits and vegetables   = +30
- ❏ I eat a combination of good and bad carbohydrate choices   = +10
- ❏ I don't eat carbs   = -20
- ❏ I eat white breads, white rice, white pasta, all kinds of sugary cereals, crackers, flour tortillas, and any carbs I can find   = -30

Total #20 = _____

21. Quality fat intake
- ❏ I consume only olive oil, canola oil, fish oil, and other unsaturated fats   = +15
- ❏ I consume good and bad fat choices   = +5
- ❏ I get my fats from butter, cheese, creams, heavy sauces, high-fat dressings, meats, and other saturated fats sources. Sat Fat is my best friend   = -15

Total #21 = _____

SAT FAT

22. Total daily dairy intake
- ❏ I don't eat or drink any dairy or dairy products like milk, cheese, yogurt, pudding, sour cream, cream cheese, or cottage cheese   = +5
- ❏ I consume some of these products, but they are usually non-fat or low-fat and I choose organic   = +5
- ❏ I consume dairy but it is not from cattle—it is from goats   = +5
- ❏ I sometimes eat or drink dairy products   = 0

❑ I like cows—so what?   = 0
❑ I eat or drink a lot of dairy and
   dairy products each day (not organic)
   —and I think Dairy Maiden is hot!   = -10
                              Total #22= _____

DAIRY MAIDEN

23. Clean calories (reading labels)
❑ I read labels and am very selective in my food choices   = +50
❑ I occasionally read labels and am somewhat selective   = +20
❑ I don't do the grocery shopping   = 0
❑ I glance at labels and know very little on this subject   = -10
❑ I don't read labels but I am kind of careful   = -20
❑ I don't read labels and I eat packaged foods quite often = -30
❑ I never read labels at all—I eat whatever I want, including
   a lot of packaged foods. I want to grow up to be just like
   Tranny Granny   = -50
                              Total #23 = _____

TRANNY GRANNY

24. Purity of calories
- Natural foods vs. processed
- Fresh foods vs. man-manipulated
- Organic vs. non-organic
- Kosher vs. non-kosher

✱ If 85% of your eating centers on one of the following sections,
mark the corresponding box:

Section A
❑ Natural, fresh, organic, and kosher foods   = +50
- Foods that are fresh and in their natural state
- Foods not manipulated by man
- Foods not packaged, frozen, canned, or processed
- If packaged, foods with 3 or fewer ingredients
- Organic always
- Foods that meet the kosher standard

Section B
- [ ] Sometimes natural, fresh, organic, and kosher foods = +20
    - Some packaged, processed foods

Section C
- [ ] Mainly packaged, frozen, and canned foods
  (which means I might end up like Mrs. Regret)   = -50
    - Many packaged, processed foods with a lot of ingredients
    —and I don't know what they are!
    - Never natural foods
    - Never fresh foods
    - Never organic
    - What does "kosher" mean?

MRS. REGRET

Section D
- [ ] Restaurant food only   = -30

* If you eat from all four sections above (which applies to most of us),
choose one of the following scores instead:
- A combination of Sections A and B   = +30
- A combination of Sections A and D   = +30
- A combination of Sections A, B, and D   = +20
- A combination of Sections B and D   = +10
- A combination of Sections B, C, and D   = -30
- A combination of Sections C and D   = -40
- A combination of Sections A, B, C, and D = You are confused, so score 0

Total #24 = _____

25. White flour intake (bread, cereals, crackers, noodles,
    pasta, pastries, tortillas, etc.)
    - [ ] I never eat any of the foods listed here   = +30
    - [ ] I eat bread and pasta only once in a while
      and they are whole grain   = +20

73

❑ I rarely eat these foods $= +10$

❑ I eat these foods once in a while $= 0$

❑ I eat all of these foods and often $= -20$

❑ These foods are my main diet and I want to hire
Mr. Bakerman to cook for me $= -30$

Total #25 = _____

MR. BAKERMAN

26. Total daily fiber intake (grams)

❑ I eat at least 25 to 35 grams of fiber every day $= +50$

❑ I eat vegetables, fruit, bran, whole grains
(like oatmeal, brown rice, and quinoa), and legumes
and nuts every day $= +20$

❑ I eat these foods a few times per week $= +5$

❑ What is fiber? $= -5$

❑ I sometimes eat these foods $= -10$

❑ I rarely to never eat from these foods $= -30$

❑ I use laxatives for my fiber $= -50$

Total #26 = _____

27. Food, sports, energy, and protein bars

❑ I rarely if ever eat food, sports, energy, or protein bars
(we'll call them "food bars") $= +15$

❑ I eat only healthy food bars with sound ingredients
(usually high in protein and fiber as well as low in fat and sugar) $= +10$

❑ I eat good-quality food bars but only in an emergency situation $= +10$

❑ I eat good-quality food bars quite often $= +5$

❑ I don't eat any food bars at all $= 0$

❑ I eat food bars but don't pay attention to their content $= -5$

❑ I choose any food bars and don't care what is in them,
even if they have 30 ingredients or more $= -15$

❑ I prefer Pop Tarts $= -15$

Total #27 = _____

28. Sauces, salad dressing, dips, and condiment intake

- ❑ I prefer my food plain   = +20
- ❑ I prefer to use olive oil, light soy sauce, mustard, salsa,
  marinara, and healthy salad dressing to sauce up my foods   = +10
- ❑ I occasionally use sauces or salad dressing but choose high-quality ones = +5
- ❑ I occasionally use sauces or salad dressing on my food
  but am not aware of the ingredients in them   = -10
- ❑ I put sauces and salad dressing on everything. (I use ketchup,
  barbecue sauce, teriyaki sauce, steak sauce, gravies, alfredo sauce—
  any type of sauce I can find—as well as all types of salad dressing)   = -15
- ❑ I prefer sauces, salad dressing, dips, and condiments to real foods   = -20

Total #28 = _____

29. Cooking and seasoning (fruits, vegetables, herbs, spices)

- ❑ I use only fruits and vegetables and fresh and untainted herbs
  and spices when I cook (like lemon, light olive oil, fresh garlic,
  basil, thyme, cilantro, oregano, and kosher sea salt, etc.)   = +15
- ❑ I don't cook, but my spouse (parents or others) does and they cook healthy
  food with fresh herbs and spices   = +10
- ❑ I don't use any type of seasoning at all (I like my food plain)   = +5
- ❑ I occasionally use teriyaki or light soy sauce or barbecue sauce to spice up meals = 0
- ❑ My cooking and seasoning habits are a combination of all of the above = -5
- ❑ I use whatever I can find to season my food   = -10
- ❑ I don't cook, but my spouse (parents or others) does and they cook
  hot dogs for me and the kids   = -15
- ❑ I mainly eat at restaurants   = -15
- ❑ I use sugar, salt, and fat when I cook (including table sugar, honey,
  molasses, and any spices that contain salt and hydrogenated fats,
  or whatever is in the product I buy)   = -15
- ❑ I used canned products to spice up my meals
  (like Hamburger Helper and Campbell's soups, etc.)   = -20
- ❑ I eat frozen TV dinners (like Lean Cuisine, Healthy Choice, etc.)   = -20

Total #29 = _____

30. Supplement intake (vitamins, minerals, and others)

- ❑ I take a multivitamin/supplement two or three times per week = +20
- ❑ I take a multivitamin/supplement once per week = +10
- ❑ I take a Flintstones vitamin when my kids do = -5
- ❑ I do have vitamins but am not good at remembering to take them = -10
- ❑ What is a multivitamin/supplement? = -20
- ❑ I take 50 pills of vitamins, fat burners, etc. = -20

Total #30 = _____

Factor #4: Restrictive and Unbalanced Dieting

31. Restrictive and unbalanced dieting

- ❑ I am on a balanced diet for my overall health & fitness = +50
  - • Protein, carbohydrates, and fats
  - • All natural, fresh, organic, and kosher foods
  - • Lean, healthy, fibrous, and alive foods
- ❑ I have never tried a restrictive or unbalanced diet = +30
- ❑ I fast occasionally for health or spiritual reasons = +20
- ❑ Sometimes I do a colon cleanse program = +15
- ❑ I am on a prescribed medical diet = +10

NURSE GIMMICK

- ✱ I can answer yes to:
- ❑ All of the following questions in this category = -50
- ❑ I tried a restrictive diet over 5 years ago = 0
- ❑ I tried a restrictive diet less than 2 years ago = -10
- ❑ I have occasionally tried restrictive diets = -20
- ❑ I have gone on many restrictive-calorie and/or unbalanced diets = -40
- ❑ I am on a restrictive diet now and I got it from Nurse Gimmick = -50
- ❑ I have taken diet pills and/or liquids to lose weight = -40
- ❑ I currently take diet pills and/or liquids to lose weight = -50
  Can I get a prescription from Dr. Pill?

DR. PILL

Total #31 = _____

Factor #5: Exercise

32. Weekly exercise program

❑ I am an athlete who trains regularly (whether
   professionally or for recreation)   = +65

❑ I do a complete and efficient exercise program
   3 to 5 times per week (it includes these 6 components)   = +50
   • Cardiovascular conditioning
   • Strength and endurance training
   • Flexibility training
   • Core and balance training
   • Corrective exercises
   • Functional training

❑ I exercise regularly 5 times per week   = +40
❑ I do a light exercise program 3 to 5 times per week = +30
❑ I will start an exercise program today   = +10
❑ I walk 3 to 5 times per week   = +10
❑ I play golf or some other sport 3 to 5 times per week = +5
❑ I walk from my bed to my car, then to the elevator,
   then home again to bed   = -20

❑ I exercise fanatically every day. I also have, will, or am
   taking performance-enhancing drugs, other "natural
   supplements," and whatever pill is on the market that
   will help me get into shape—no matter what. I want to
   be just like George   = -30

GEORGE GOTTA GO

❑ What is exercise?   = -30
❑ I play video games for my exercise   = -40
❑ I hate to exercise and I never will. I want to be
   just as lazy as Vegg   = -65

Total #32 = _____

End of quiz.

VEGG

STOP. Review the quiz to make sure you have answered all the questions
and chosen only one response for each.

Diva Diet Quiz Scores

- Copy your score from each numbered Quiz question and write it below in the corresponding space.
- Add up your points for each of the Five Factors for a factor total.
- Add up all your factor totals for a final total Diva Diet Quiz Score.

Factor #1: Liquid Consumption

1. Water   Score: _____
2. Coffee and other caffeinated drinks   Score: _____
3. Tea   Score: _____
4. Soda   Score: _____
5. Other drinks   Score: _____
6. Juice   Score: _____
7. Meal replacement drinks   Score: _____
8. Alcohol   Score: _____

Factor #1 total: _____

Factor #2: Quality and Distribution of Daily Calories

9. Daily caloric intake   Score: _____
10. Daily nutrient ratio: protein/carbs/fat   Score: _____
11. Number of meals per day   Score: _____
12. Meal timing   Score: _____
13. Meal size   Score: _____

Factor #2 total: _____

Factor #3: Quality and Purity of Calories

14. Junk food   Score: _____
15. Total daily fat intake   Score: _____

16. Total daily sugar intake   Score: _____
17. Sugar substitutes intake   Score: _____
18. Total daily sodium intake   Score: _____
19. Quality protein intake   Score: _____
20. Quality carbohydrate intake   Score: _____
21. Quality fat intake   Score: _____
22. Total daily dairy intake   Score: _____
23. Clean calories   Score: _____
24. Purity of calories   Score: _____
25. White flour intake   Score: _____
26. Total daily fiber intake   Score: _____
27. Food, sports, energy, and protein bars   Score: _____
28. Sauces, salad dressing, dips, and condiment intake   Score: _____
29. Cooking and seasoning   Score: _____
30. Supplement intake   Score: _____

Factor #3 total: _____

Factor #4: Restrictive and Unbalanced Dieting

31. Restrictive and unbalanced diets

Factor #4 total: _____

Factor #5: Exercise

32. Weekly exercise program

Factor #5 total: _____

Add up all your factor totals here: _____

Subtract 35 points to adjust for estimate errors: — 35

Diva Diet Quiz Total Real Score = _____

Diva Diet Quiz Grades

Paw Body Fat Rating Guide

Body Fat %	Diva Rating
10 to 15% body fat and below	Athletic (exceptional)
16 to 19% body fat	Extra-low body fat (excellent)
20 to 21% body fat	Low body fat (very good)
22% body fat	Good shape (good)
23 to 25% body fat	High body fat (poor)
26 to 34% body fat	Very high body fat (unhealthy)
35% body fat and up	Extra-high body fat (deficient)

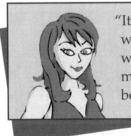

"It's not what you weigh—it's all about what the pounds are made of: fat or lean body mass."

A = 541 to 830

- If you scored in this range (especially in the 700 to 800 range), you should already have low body fat (below 20%) and be in great shape, with phenomenal health (you may even consider writing your own diet program!).

- Are you a nutritionist or fitness expert with great health and low body fat (below 20%)? Thanks for reading our book. We hope you tell your friends about MY DIVA DIET.

- Maybe you hired a true fitness professional to help you eat right and exercise. Congratulations—again, you should be very healthy & fit.

- If you scored an A and are eating well but still have high body fat (over 25%), then maybe you are not exercising enough. If you begin a regular exercise program, you should make immediate progress.

B = 301 to 540

- Scoring in this range is great and means you are already in good shape (around 22% body fat) and have good health. Keep it up!
- With just a few adjustments in your overall diet plan, you can get in excellent shape (16 to 19% fat or even less) and experience even better health.

If you scored an A or B and still have high body fat (over 25%), make sure you have answered each question honestly and have accurately calculated your totals. If you have answered accurately and you are already on a good exercise program, then tighten up on those areas of your diet where you need improvement—you will lose fat.

C = 0 to 300

- Scoring in this range means you are average in your overall diet regimen: Your eating habits aren't great, but they're not terrible either.
- You won't have to get ultra-strict with your diet plan, but you will have to change. If you improve your eating habits, you can rest assured that less body fat and good health are on their way.
- Make sure your exercise program is appropriate.
- Being average is good news, but you still need to consider your body fat and overall health. If you want to become healthier and more fit, now is the time to make changes.

D = -1 to -430

- A score in this category means that your eating habits are not good but they are not drastically bad either—at least not yet. With the right adjustments to your diet and a good exercise program, you will get results.
- If you are already in good shape here despite eating poorly, then you have a great metabolism and you will get leaner quickly. You can easily get into great shape (22% fat and below). But, it would be interesting to find out what your overall health is really like.

- Even if you scored in this range and have a higher body fat (closer to 27 to 30% or even 35% and above), you will get results if you begin to change your eating habits and either start or perfect your exercise program (unless you are a chronic yo-yo dieter).

F = -431 to -875

- If you score here, we have only one question for you—what are you eating?
- The good news is that with some adjustments in your diet and adding an exercise routine you will be able to lose fat immediately.
- A warning: make sure you get a full physical evaluation prior to beginning a diet or exercise program, because if you are eating this poorly, you may have some health problems brewing and not know it.

If you're a woman scoring in the D and F ranges, you actually will see fast results unless some of the following conditions exist:
- You are a chronic yo-yo dieter
- You are just coming off a starvation or restrictive diet
- You are just coming off diet pills
- You have a metabolic problem
- You are on medications that inhibit fat loss

If you're a woman scoring in the A and B ranges, yet you still have high body fat, you may initially have more difficulty in reaching your low body fat goals. But, with perseverance, you will accomplish them.

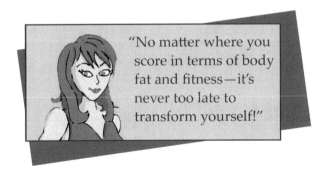

"No matter where you score in terms of body fat and fitness—it's never too late to transform yourself!"

For a more in-depth picture of your eating and exercise habits, transfer your Five Factor subtotals and final Diva Diet Quiz Score to Worksheet #2 (Diva Diet Quiz Summary and The Five Factors Scores) in PART EIGHT (pages 352-355). There you can review how you did within each of the Five Factors and get to know and target your Diet Villains.

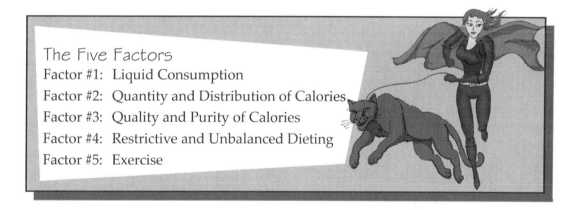

The Five Factors
Factor #1: Liquid Consumption
Factor #2: Quantity and Distribution of Calories
Factor #3: Quality and Purity of Calories
Factor #4: Restrictive and Unbalanced Dieting
Factor #5: Exercise

"Wherever you are now, MY DIVA DIET can help you:
• Lose fat—gain health
• Fix a factor
• Defeat the Diet Villains
• Learn more about diet and exercise
• Prevent high body fat and poor health!"

PART FOUR

The Guidelines

A wise man (woman) will hear and increase learning.
And a man of understanding will attain wise counsel.

-Proverbs 1:5

The Five Factors: Notes, Rules, and FYI's

In PART FOUR we provide you with some background information on the thirty-two sub-topics of the Five Factors Affecting Body Fat and Health (the thirty-two question categories you responded to in PART THREE's Diva Diet Quiz). We also give you some MY DIVA DIET rules that will help you get healthy & fit for life.

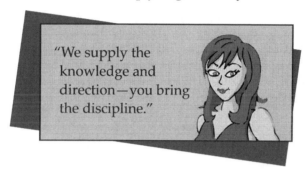

"We supply the knowledge and direction—you bring the discipline."

Our summaries in this section apply to both phases of the MY DIVA DIET—the Diva Reduction Phase and the Diva Maintenance Phase—as indicated.

Factor #1: Liquid Consumption

1. Water

Water is essential for life—it makes up about two-thirds of a person's body weight and is the second most important nutrient next to oxygen. We can live without food for weeks, but only a few days without water. Drinking plenty of water stands alone as the best thing you can do for your body.

* Notes
- Water is critical to good health.
  - Water is necessary for nearly every bodily function, including circulation, digestion, absorption, excretion, and nutrient distribution to all cells.
  - Adequate amounts of water are vital to lung function; mitigate high blood pressure, high cholesterol levels, obesity, diabetes, asthma, gastrointestinal problems, hiatal hernias, headaches, angina, allergies, and constipation; prevent kidney stones; and slow aging.

- Lack of water can affect our weight-loss efforts.
  - Most of us retain water because we do not drink enough water.
  - We mistake thirst for hunger, so we eat instead of drinking water.
  - Dehydration not only has health consequences but also affects our mood and can make us lethargic, making it impossible to exercise and eat correctly.
- Thirst cannot always be relied on as the best indicator of water requirements. If you're thirsty, you're probably already dehydrated.

✱ Water Rules
- Supply your body with enough water each day and you will reap the rewards of health, vitality, energy, great skin, appetite control, reduced fat and bloating, and much more.
- Drink an average of eight to ten cups of water or more each day (depending on your body weight).
  - You may need more water if you are exercising, drinking coffee or other caffeinated drinks, taking medications, and/or drinking alcohol.
  - You will get some water from your consumption of whole grains, fruits, vegetables, and some liquids you consume each day.
- It's best to drink room-temperature water—iced water can delay digestion if consumed with a meal.

✱ FYI's
- Drinking bottled water is probably better than drinking tap water, unless you do enough research to be confident that your tap water is being properly treated and is safe.
- Another option is a tap-water filtering system, which is much less expensive than bottled water.

2. Coffee and other caffeinated drinks

If you think that just because you don't drink coffee or you drink decaf that you aren't consuming any caffeine, think again. Under current federal regulations a product labeled "decaffeinated" can still contain 2.5% of the original amount of caffeine, and caffeine is also found in tea, soda, energy drinks, chocolate, candy, medications, and diet pills.

❋ Notes
- Coffee itself is not the problem so much as is consuming too much caffeine.
  - Caffeine acts as a stimulant and can cause your heart to pump faster and your breathing to quicken.
  - Caffeine acts as a diuretic, which increases the body's need for more water.
  - Caffeine is also a drug that can be addictive, so people who consume caffeine every day will usually need to continue to consume the same amount of caffeine just to feel normal.

❋ Coffee and Other Caffeinated Drink Rules
- Coffee is okay in moderation, especially without sugar and cream.
  - A little honey or agave nectar is good for sweetening coffee, as is low-fat milk because of its lactose (milk sugar) content.
  - Skip dry creamers—they contain hydrogenated oil as well as sugar and other unwholesome ingredients—try a little low-fat soy milk or rice milk instead.
- Watch out for those fancy coffee drinks—they are full of fat and sugar.
- Tea is a good substitute for coffee—it's low in caffeine and has other beneficial qualities.
- Avoid soda—not just because of the caffeine but for other reasons as well (see Soda, #4).
- Be cautious of so-called "energy drinks", as they usually contain high amounts of caffeine.
- Chocolate is okay on occasion, but choose dark chocolate instead of milk or white.
- Be aware of caffeine in medications you are taking.
- Stay away from diet pills!

❋ FYI's
- Coffee beans are produced by the *Coffea* plant, a small evergreen plant. Once ripe, coffee berries are picked, processed, and dried, then roasted to varying degrees (depending on desired flavor) and brewed for coffee.
- It's been suggested that coffee may provide health benefits because of its antioxidants, which help prevent free radicals from causing cell damage.
- Coffee's negative health effects are mostly due to excessive consumption of the caffeine it contains, which research suggests may create temporary problems such as increase in the stiffening of arterial walls, magnesium deficiency, and a mixed effect on short-term memory.

The following chart (provided at Starbucks stores or online at www.starbucks.com/nutrition) shows a breakdown of common Starbucks coffee drinks ("Grande" size—16 fluid ounces, except where noted).

LIQUID CHART

Drink	Calories	Fat (g)	Sodium (mg)	Sugar (g)	Caffeine (mg)	Carbs (g)
Coffee (plain)	5	0	10	0	330	0
Espresso (1 oz.)	5	0	0	0	75	1
Café Latte (low fat)	190	7	150	17	150	18
Cappuccino (low fat)	120	4	85	10	150	12
Café Mocha (whole milk, no whipped cream)	290	12	120	31	175	40
White Chocolate Mocha (whole milk, with whipped cream)	500	22	240	59	150	62
Mocha Frappuccino	380	15	240	57	115	47
Whipped cream only *	80	8	10	2	0	2

* Whipped cream ingredients (store bought): Cream, nonfat milk, corn syrup, sugar, mono- and diglycerides, natural and artificial flavors, carrageenan, and propellant (nitrous oxide)

3. Tea

After water, tea is the most commonly consumed beverage in the world, offering many health benefits if you skip the cream and sugar. The average amount of caffeine in tea is 40 milligrams per cup, compared to coffee, which contains around 100 milligrams per cup.

* Notes
• Teas such as green, black, and red contain polyphenols, which are rich in antioxidants that help protect our bodies from free radical damage and may reduce the risk of gastric, esophageal, and skin cancers.

- Polyphenols also help prevent blood clotting, lower cholesterol levels, and may lower the risk of ovarian cancer.
- Herbal teas are infusions made with herbs, flowers, spices, roots. and other plant parts but do not have the same health-promoting properties as green, red, and black teas. Herbal teas are consumed for their physical or medicinal effects, especially for their digestive, immunity, cleansing, relaxant, and wellness properties.

✶ Tea Rules
- Drink a couple of cups of tea daily to help boost your water intake and add other health benefits. With such a wide variety of flavors you're bound to find one or more you love.
- Don't drink grocery store or convenience store bottled teas that aren't 100% tea.

  These teas usually contain sugar, high fructose corn syrup, and other sugar derivatives, all of which are definite no-no's.
  - Try pre-made unsweetened Tejava tea (www.tejava.com), found at Trader Joe's.
- Some coffee bistros offer a variety of tea choices—just make sure they are plain teas—no sugar, cream, artificial sweeteners, etc..

4. Soda

Americans are drinking more soda today than ever before—soft drinks account for more than 25% of all drinks consumed.

✶ Notes
- Drinking soda contributes to four major health issues: obesity, tooth decay, weakened bones, and caffeine dependence.
- Soda and other soft drinks are not healthy for you, even when they are labeled "decaffeinated" or "diet."

✶ Soda Rule
- MY DIVA DIET recommends avoiding soda because its lack of nutritional value, adverse health effects, addictive quality, and contribution to weight gain.

✶ FYI's
- If you've analyzed one soda, you've analyzed most of them.
  - Regular sodas are made up of carbonated water, high fructose corn syrup, citric acid or phosphoric acid, and other natural flavors.

- Many diet sodas contain carbonated water, caramel color, aspartame, phosphoric acid, potassium benzoate, natural flavors, citric acid, and caffeine.
- Other diet sodas contain carbonated water, phosphoric acid, sugar or high fructose corn syrup, aspartame, acesulfame-k, and sucralose.
- Some diet sodas contain Splenda or other artificially made sweeteners.
- Most regular and diet sodas contain caffeine.

LIQUID CHART

Soda (8oz.)	Calories	Sugar (g)	Sodium (mg)	Caffeine (mg)
Diet Coke	0	0	40	30.4
Diet Pepsi	0	0	25	24
Coke/Pepsi	100	27	35	23
Sprite	100	26	45	0

5. Other drinks (sports drinks, powdered soft drinks, juice boxes, and other sugary drinks)

Sports drinks are made up of water, sugar, and maybe a few vitamins. Most juices and drinks labeled "juice" are mainly water, sugar, and a splash of juice.

* Notes

- Powdered soft drinks and juice boxes are packed with either sugar or artificial sweeteners.
- Most, if not all, of these drinks are primarily water and sugar (high fructose corn syrup, sucrose syrup, and glucose-fructose syrup), plus other ingredients.
- Just like soda, the drinks in this category labeled "diet" contain artificially made sweeteners.
  - These are unnecessary calories and potentially harmful ingredients and chemicals added to your daily diet.
  - Sugar is easily converted into body fat.
- If you are an athlete or if you exercise vigorously, then sports drinks may be of use to you if they have been properly evaluated and are being monitored.

* Other Drink Rules
- Sports drinks, powdered soft drinks, juice boxes, and other sugary drinks are not recommended on MY DIVA DIET.
  - Sports drinks and vitamin waters may be the exception, as some contain vitamins and minerals.
- Water remains the best fluid to put in your body.
  - If you need flavor in your water, try adding fresh fruit like lemon, strawberries, or pineapple.

* FYI"s
The following table lists some common drinks with a breakdown of calories, sugar, and sodium.

LIQUID CHART

Name	Calories	Sugar (g)	Sodium (mg)	Nutritional Value
Orange juice (8 oz.)	110	22	0	Vitamin C and traces of other vitamins
Cranberry juice from concentrate (8 oz.)	130	33	35	35 mg potassium
Snapple (8 oz.)	50	12	5	No
Lemonade (not fresh/ sugar added) (8 oz.)	110	27	40	No
Capri Sun (6.75 oz.)	90	24	15	No
Sports waters				
Gatorade (8 oz.)	90	22	160	Some
Propel (8 oz.)	10	2	35	Traces of vitamins C, E, niacin, B_6, B_{12}, pantothenic acid
Vitamin Water (8 oz.)	50	13	0	Some vitamins (depending on flavor)
SoBe Life Water (8 oz.)	50	13	0	A lot of vitamin C, traces of E, niacin, B_6, B_{12}, pantothenic acid

6. Juice (fruit and vegetable): fresh vs. concentrated

Drinking juice (unless it is fresh and from real fruits and vegetables in their natural form) is another way we unknowingly add excessive calories to our diet.

✱ Notes
- Most commercial juices:
  - Contain large amounts of sugar
  - Contain very little of the fruit or vegetable they are supposedly derived from
  - Contain little, if any, nutritional value
  - Are very high in calories and low in fiber—the opposite of most fruits and vegetables in their natural complete states
- Fruit and vegetable juices are not as beneficial as whole fruits and vegetables because:
  - The entire fruit or vegetable is not used. The outer layers of fruits and vegetables are full of vitamins, minerals, antioxidants, fiber, and other nutrients, and these are usually not used in juicing.
  - In order to make one cup of a fruit or vegetable juice, you probably have to use at least five to ten pieces of that particular fruit or vegetable. This means five or more times the total calories.

✱ Juice Rules
- The only way fruit and vegetable juices are of any benefit is if they are fresh and all parts (including the skin when possible) are used. You can ensure this by using a proper juicer (Jack LaLanne makes a very good one).
- If you do buy juice, always read the labels and look for 100% juice, not juice from concentrate.
  - Fresh juice without preservatives usually has a short shelf life—check expiration dates.
  - Try plain cranberry juice diluted in water!

7. Meal replacement drinks (protein shakes, smoothies, and green drinks)

In today's society we gravitate toward anything that is quick and easy, and this also holds true for replacing healthful meals with quick drinks.

* Notes
- The billion-dollar fitness industry makes its money off quick-fix scams and false promises. Next time you pick up a so-called "diet shake," "protein shake," "energy drink," or "vegetable drink," take a look at the ingredients.
    - Most of these drinks (if they are pre-made) contain large amounts of sugar as well as preservatives and additives.
    - The protein used is questionable, as are some of the claims being made.

* Meal Replacement Drink Rules
- Meal replacement drinks can be an acceptable way to get nutrients on the run.
    - If they are of good quality, these types of drinks are okay to use as a meal, especially if you are pressed for time. They are much better solutions than skipping a meal or grabbing a high-fat donut or muffin.
    - Meal replacement drinks can also be used as supplements to ensure that you get all the nutrients you need each day for optimal health & fitness.
- The best advice in this area is to know what is in a pre-made protein shake, smoothie, or green (or other vegetable) drink.
- Best of all, you can make these drinks yourself using real foods without added ingredients.
    - When making your own protein shake, smoothie, or green drink at home, use real juice, fruits, nuts, flaxseed, bran, yogurt, etc.
        - For protein shakes, use a protein powder blend that has low amounts of sugar and no additives. There are many good ones to choose from , and they are a good way to ensure you get enough protein without sacrificing quality.
- Many health food stores, fitness centers, and other places include these drinks on their menus—just ask questions.
    - Try your local juice bar, like Jamba Juice (www.jambajuice.com).

* FYI's
- Here are some different types of protein powders and basic information about each:
    - Whey protein is the most commonly used type of protein. It contains high levels of essential amino acids.
    - Casein protein powder is the richest in glutamine, an amino acid that aids in recovery.
    - Egg white protein is a lactose- and dairy-free protein.

- Soy protein contains all the amino acids and is a good alternative for vegetarians.
- Hemp protein contains essential amino acids and is another good vegetarian alternative.
- Green and other vegetable drinks are a great way to supplement our diets because it is often difficult to eat all the nutrients we need each day, especially when it comes to vegetables. Some green drinks are loaded with vitamins, minerals, and antioxidants. Some even contain amino acids, herbs, probiotics, enzymes, and fiber. You just have to make sure of the quality and watch the ingredients.
  - Here are some excellent products for making a quick and healthful green drink:
    - Living Fuel (www.livingfuel.com)
    - Garden of Life Perfect Food (www.gardenoflife.com)
    - Energy First Green Energy Super Food (www.energyfirst.com)
    - Bolthouse Farms—a pre-made green drink you can find in your grocery or health food store (www.bolthouse.com)

8. Alcohol

The behavioral problems that can result from alcohol use and abuse are well documented. However, alcohol consumption also has a direct impact on your health as well as your body-fat level.

✱ Notes
- Alcohol has short-term effects on health and body fat.
  - Alcohol is easily converted to fat, has empty calories, can cause dehydration, and creates electrolyte imbalances.
  - While your liver is busy metabolizing alcohol, it is unable to metabolize fat.
- Alcohol has more severe long-term effects on health and body fat.
  - Excessive alcohol use can result in dependency, nutrition deficiency (mainly B-complex and iron), liver dysfunction, brain cell damage, increased cancer risk, increased heart disease risk, digestive system dysfunction, reproductive problems, and mental health effects (like depression).

✱ Alcohol Rules
- If you are serious about losing fat and upgrading your health, alcohol has to be off limits during the Diva Reduction Phase of MY DIVA DIET.

- When you are in the Diva Maintenance Phase, you can have alcohol in moderation, but you will need to monitor it so that the fat does not come back and your health won't suffer.

✱ FYI's
- The following chart shows you the average caloric content of some common alcoholic drinks.

LIQUID CHART	
Drink	**Calories**
Wine (4 oz.)	90
One beer (12 oz.)	150 to 200 (depending on brand)
Bloody Mary	115 calories
Whiskey sour	122
Gin and tonic	171
Piña colada	262
Vodka / other alcohol (4 oz.)	250 (depending on choice)

Calories from wine, beer, alcohol, alcoholic mixed drinks (the mix adds an additional 100+ calories) add up quickly—a few drinks can total up to one half of your daily calories or more.

Factor #2: Quantity and Distribution of Calories

9. Daily caloric intake (overeating or undereating)
How many calories are you consuming per day? What are your eating patterns?

✱ Notes
- We are a country in which half of our citizens—and 31 to 38% of our children—are obese, primarily because we just eat too much. In fact, when it comes to food, we are a nation of extremes, either overeating or starving ourselves to lose weight.
- We super-size everything—except water! Most of the food we eat has almost no nutritional value and contributes to fat storage and health issues like obesity, high blood pressure, high cholesterol levels, certain cancers, etc.

- Some of us eat too much:
  - We start our day with coffee and orange juice and maybe a piece of toast. Or we stop at a drive-through and order a big breakfast burrito.
  - At lunch we order fast food.
  - At 5 p.m. we find ourselves at "Happy Hour" (by this time we have already consumed 2,000 calories).
  - At dinner we eat a big plate of steak and potatoes (after a salad and five pieces of bread with butter). Now our calorie count is up to 4,000 and we're starting to think about dessert.
- Some of us eat too little:
  - We skip breakfast or gulp down a Slim-Fast.
  - We skip lunch or just have a salad.
  - By mid-afternoon we're tired and grumpy because our calorie level is at 200.
    - We may buy one of those high-fat, high-sugar coffee drinks or a high-caffeine energy drink to solve our fatigue problem, which only results in a surge and then a drop in energy an hour later.
    - We may also sneak in a protein bar or piece of fruit.
  - By dinnertime we are famished, so we eat anything and everything we can find.
    - Maybe we have a frozen dinner. We decide on a "healthy" diet frozen dinner. We think we are doing ourselves a favor, but there is nothing "healthy," "lean," or "smart" about this kind of choice.
  - At the end of the day we congratulate ourselves for having consumed only 800 calories, but in fact we have failed to nourish our bodies properly and have probably eaten a variety of actively harmful foods.
- Our third problem eating pattern is not eating all day until nighttime, when we are so hungry that we quickly consume 3,000 calories at once. Not only have we been unproductive during the day, but we are now over-full. This habit is very unhealthy, causing weight gain and lethargy.

✱ Daily Caloric Intake Rules
- The average woman should consume between 1,200 and 1,600 calories per day.
  - A woman can and should consume more than 1,600 if she has a high metabolism, or is an athlete, pregnant, or has a medical condition that warrants a higher caloric intake.
  - Young girls and women trying to gain weight also need more calories.

- Anything over 3,000 calories per day is not a good idea unless we are athletes or have some sort of medical condition.
- Anything under 1,000 calories per day is considered starvation and will cause the body to go into survival mode—hold on to body fat not release it!. Undereating will not only hinder the body's ability to get fit, but it will also jeopardize health.

✱ FYI's
- Figuring out how many calories we should eat each day is somewhat complex and has many variables.
  - Daily caloric intake is calculated according to BMR, lean body mass, age, activity level, gender, and weight-management goals.
  - Medical conditions are always a factor in determining daily calories.
  - Another consideration when calculating daily calories is whether you are interested in losing body fat, gaining muscle, or just maintaining your current condition.
  - Our lifestyles have to be taken into consideration as well, including whether or not we exercise.
  - A final factor to consider is if you've just ended a long period of starvation or restrictive-type dieting, or you have been taking diet pills.

10. Daily nutrient ratio: protein/carbohydrates/fat

- "Nutritious" means "contributing to health or growth"
- "Nutrient" means "a nutritious ingredient or substance in a food"
- "Essential nutrient" means "a nutrient required for the health and growth of an organism but not synthesized in the body"

Proper nutrition requires a balance of all essential nutrients. To deny ourselves any one nutrient is to ask for trouble. The tricky part, as described above, is to find out which daily caloric intake and nutrient balance is right for you.

✱ Notes
- Any time you restrict or are missing nutrients from one of the three main categories—protein, carbohydrates, and fat—you put your health & fitness at risk. That's why these nutrients are referred to as "essential."
- Most nutrition experts, dieticians, and fitness gurus agree that we need to eat foods from all three groups, but there is always a debate about the exact numbers.

* Daily Nutrient Ratio Rules
- Calories in a healthy and fit diet should come from all three categories of essential nutrients: protein, carbohydrates, and fat. MY DIVA DIET recommends the following:

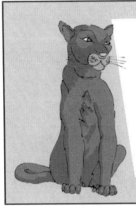

Paw Nutrient Ratio Guide

Diva Reduction Phase:
35% protein/45% carbs/20% fat (or close)

Diva Maintenance Phase:
20 to 35% protein/45 to 65% carbs/20 to 30% fat *

   * Maintenance ratio can fluctuate

   * Extra-lean Divas can go as low as 15% fat

- For a 1,300-calorie day during the Diva Reduction Phase, your breakdown of nutrients (in grams) would look like this:

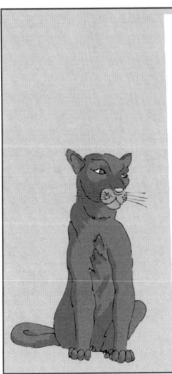

Paw Daily Nutrient Guide
Protein—Carbs—Fat

Diva Reduction Phase
Daily Nutrient Ratio =
35% protein/45%carbs/20%fat

Standard 1,300 Calories Per Day
- Protein = 113.8 grams
- Carbs = 146.3 grams
- Fat = 28.9 grams

Preferred Daily Range
- Protein = 100 to 120 grams
- Carbs = 130 to 150 grams
- Fat = 25 to 30 grams
- Fiber = 25 to 35 grams

* FYI's
- Consider planning an "all-vegetarian day" once a month. Skip meats, poultry, fish, eggs, and dairy—focus on eating legumes, nuts, grains, fruits, and vegetables. You will feel truly refreshed.

11. Number of meals per day (including snacks)

There is another way we miss the mark. We think we are doing ourselves a favor by not eating all day, but by dinnertime we are starving and we overeat, grabbing whatever is at hand—and most of the time that "convenient" food is not healthy or fit.

* Notes
- When we are trying to become or stay healthy & fit, we want our calories to be used rather than stored as fat. More calories are stored as fat when we eat too much at one sitting.
  - Glycogen storage—complex carbohydrates stored in the liver and muscles for later energy use—is okay, as long as we don't store too much.
- We also need to watch our blood glucose levels.
  - When we eat small, healthy, and fit meals every three or four hours, we can keep our blood glucose level stable, thus avoiding highs and lows in blood sugar.
  - A stable blood glucose level will also help us burn fat more efficiently throughout the day.
  - Eating frequent small meals is a much better safeguard for controlling blood glucose levels than relying solely on the glycemic index—a way of ranking carbohydrates according to their effect on blood glucose levels.

* Number of Meals Per Day Rules
- Take your 1,200 to 1,600 (or more) calories and break them down into four to five meals evenly spaced throughout the day, including snacks. For example, a 1,200-calorie day would mean 300 calories per meal.

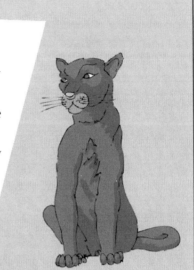

Paw Daily Meal Plan Quick Guide

- Try to eat quality protein in 2 or 3 of your daily meals.
- Eat quality carbs in all 4 meals (just watch the type and amount).
- The fat will fall into place. (Fat is found in many protein-rich foods, and traces are found in grains, fruits, and vegetables.)
  - Keep added fat to a minimum.
- Don't forget your fiber.

* FYI's
- Here are a few tips to help you eat frequent small meals evenly spaced throughout the day for beneficial fat loss, health, and overall well-being:
  - Plan ahead—cook more in the evening so you will have food for your breakfast and lunch the next day.
    - Keep freshly cut vegetables available for snacks, to include in your lunch, for tortilla wrap and sandwich meals, and for omelets, soups, salads, etc.
    - Pack your own lunch (and some snacks) for the day—it's a great way to control your food choices.
- Glass or ceramic containers for food storage are preferable to disposable plastic containers.
  - Some health experts are concerned that plastic containers may release carcinogenic toxins into foods.

12. Meal timing
Meal timing is another area that can make or break us when it comes to fat loss, productivity, and feeling good.

* Notes
- Eating healthy meals early in the day enables the body and brain to function properly, and will guarantee that calories are used for their intended purpose.

- Eating too much late at night is a good way to fail at losing those unwanted fat pounds—and could be one of the habits that led to weight gain in the first place.

✱ Meal Timing Rules
- Time your meals according to your own wake-up and bedtime schedule.
- Try to eat every three to four hours.
- Eat larger meals early in the day and keep evening meals light to ensure that your calories are used for health and energy and not stored as fat.
    - The exception to late-night eating applies to those who work late at night. Just try to eat your last meal three hours prior to going to bed.

13. Meal size (portion control)

This is another enormous problem in the American diet. If you are eating until you feel overly full, you are adding to your weight problems. You can only assimilate so many nutrients at one time—as noted above, the rest are stored as fat.

✱ Notes
- We need to concentrate on the amount of food on our plates. We need nourishment, but not 2,000 calories at one sitting.
- We need to learn when to stop eating.

✱ Meal Size Rules
- Here are four portion control tips:
    #1   Stop eating so much.
    #2   Stop super-sizing everything.
    #3   Don't keep eating just because everyone else is.
    #4   Exercise self-control!
- Feeling full helps you decide when you've had enough food, but it's not always the best gauge to help you stop eating.
    - Try ending a meal three to five bites before you actually begin to feel full.
- Feeling full after drinking water would be the only exception here.

✱ FYI's
- The following pages provide some helpful tools to clarify portion control:

Paw Recommended Calories Guide
(Per Meal)

Daily Caloric Intake	Maximum Calories Per Meal
1,200 calories	300
1,300 calories	325
1,400 calories	350
1,600 calories	400

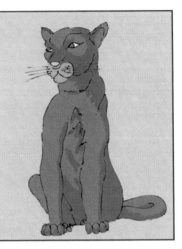

Paw Common Foods Portion Guide
(Per Meal)

Category	Diva Portion Size (Reduction Phase to Maintenance Phase)
• Protein (Animal)	
Beef, poultry, fish	3 to 5 oz. (cooked)
Egg whites	2 to 6
Whole eggs	1 to 2
• Dairy and dairy products	
Milk, yogurt, cottage cheese	1/2 to 1 cup
Sour cream, cream cheese	1/2 to 2 Tbsp.
Parmesan cheese	1 to 2 Tbsp.
Cheese, butter	1 to 2 oz.
• Protein (Plant)	
Legumes	1/2 to 1-1/2 cup
Nuts, seeds	1 to 3 oz.
• Carbohydrates	
Whole grains	1/2 to 1-1/2 cup (cooked)
Breads, tortillas, etc.	1 to 2 slices
Pasta	1/2 to 1-1/2 cup (cooked)
Rice and corn cakes	1 to 5 whole
Cereals	1/2 to 1-1/2 cup
Fruits	1 to 3 whole (except avocados)
Vegetables	1 to 3 cups
• Fats	
Oils, salad dressing, sauces	1 to 2 Tbsp.
Spreads (nut butter, mayonnaise, etc.)	1 tsp to 2 Tbsp.
• Other	
Sweeteners (honey, agave nectar)	1 tsp to 2 Tbsp.

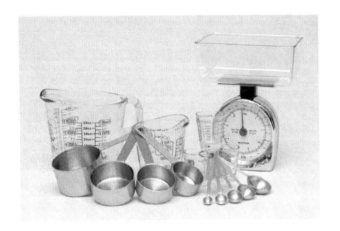

Portion control tools: Measuring cups, bowls, and spoons will help you when you begin tracking portion sizes. After you use them for a while, you will be able to estimate amounts on sight. A food scale is also helpful.

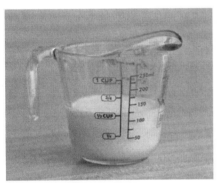

1/2 cup milk

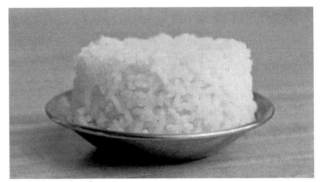

1 cup cooked rice

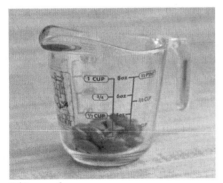

1/4 cup legumes

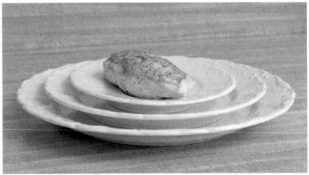

4 oz. cooked chicken breast

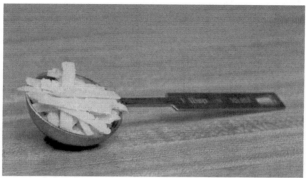

1 Tbsp. Parmesan cheese

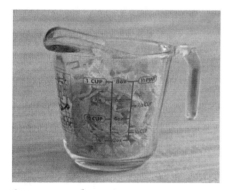

1 cup cereal

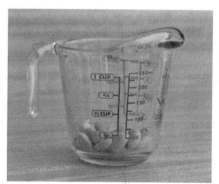

1/4 cup nuts

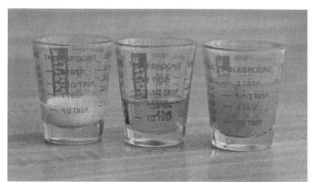

1/2 Tbsp. - 1 Tbsp. olive oil and 2 Tbsp.
salad dressing

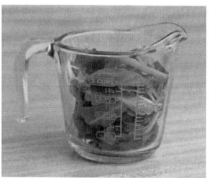

2 cups vegetables

Factor #3: Quality and Purity of Calories

14. Junk food (fast food, pizza, ice cream, potato chips, cookies, candy, donuts, etc.)

Junk food makes up about 50% or more of today's American diet, and many people lack an understanding of how its prevalence affects body fat and health issues. MY DIVA DIET wants you to know that junk food is just what its name implies, and it underlies many of our worst food choices, wreaks havoc on our health, and is a major factor in our obesity epidemic.

* Notes
- Junk food goes far beyond candy, cake, donuts, and commonly prepared desserts:
  - It comprises most fast food.
  - It includes soda and other sugary drinks.
  - It also comprises many of the packaged, processed, and refined foods so popular today, including but not limited to crackers and snack items, frozen and canned foods, cereals, etc.
  - It also includes items made with hidden flour, sugar, sodium, and fake fats.
  - It incorporates many foods that are man-made, especially wholesome foods that are:
    - Manipulated in any form
    - Made with artificial ingredients
    - Packed full of preservatives and additives

* Junk Food Rules
- In general, stay away from fast food and the other junk food items listed above, as well as the ones you already know about.
- Be cautious and extremely selective when choosing man-made food products—less is better here.
- Eating junk food once in a while might be okay, but some choices are better than others.
  - Do a little research: in addition to reading labels, check some of the charts available on restaurant menus and at fast-food eating places.
- There are much better choices than junk food when you want dessert or just a sweet treat, such as frozen yogurt, sorbet, pudding, and gluten-free fig bars.

＊ FYI's

• The following is a list of just a few junk food items that are consumed regularly. At first glance, you may think some of them are low in calories or fat, but when you read their ingredient panels you'll discover that most contain anywhere from twenty to seventy-five items, including trans fats, sugar, flavor enhancers, preservatives, MSG, white and wheat flour, milk, nuts, cheese cultures, and other unwholesome ingredients.

  • Even when trans fats are omitted (a recent trend), these foods contain saturated fat and other harmful ingredients.

  • Most of these types of foods (including the fat-free products) do not have any fiber or nutritional value.

FOOD CHART

Product	Calories	Protein (g)	Carbs (g)	Fat (g)	Sugar (g)	Sodium (mg)
Potato chips (1 oz.)	160	1	14	11	1	170
Fruit snacks (1 roll)	50	0	12	1	7	55
Cookies (3 chocolate chip, reduced fat)	140	2	23	5	11	150
Donuts (4 mini)	240	1.2	15.5	4.6	16	240
Lemon cake (1 slice, 3 oz.)	130	2	19	9	11	105
Cheese 'n Crackers	100	2	10	5	2	340
Cheetos (1 small bag)	160	2	15	10	1	290
Cheezit (25 mini crackers)	150	2	18	8	0	280
Chex Mix (2/3 cup)	130	2	22	4	2	380
100-calorie snacks	100	2	12	6	1	6

15. Total daily fat intake (grams)

Total fat intake is a major factor in our obesity epidemic and many other health issues. That is why food companies started producing "fat-free" foods in the 1980s and '90s. Yet we are still fat. Why? Mainly because we consume too many processed and man-made foods instead of fresh foods in their natural states, we switched from fat to sugar, and we also switched to foods containing trans fats and hydrogenated oils.

✳ Notes

- There are five areas to address in any discussion of fats: polyunsaturated, monounsaturated, and saturated fats; cholesterol; and trans-fatty acids (hydrogenated fats).
  - Polyunsaturated fats, unlike saturated fats, are beneficial to your health.
    - These fats help prevent heart disease by lowering blood cholesterol levels and help to reduce arthritis and other joint problems and some skin diseases.
    - These fats are found in sources like oily fish and cooking oils like safflower, grapeseed, sunflower, and corn.
  - Monounsaturated fats are now thought by some experts to have health benefits as well, such as reducing heart disease risk.
    - These fats are found in sources like olives, olive oil, nuts, and avocados.
  - Saturated fats are found in sources like meat and meat products, dairy, and coconut oil and other tropical oils.
    - These fats should be kept to a minimum—they are known to increase health risks by causing a rise in blood cholesterol levels, which can lead to heart disease.
  - Cholesterol is found in certain animal foods (meat, poultry, shellfish, egg yolks, and dairy products) and in some man-made food products.
    - The body makes its own cholesterol, so we really do not need to consume much in our daily diet.
  - Trans-fatty acids are found in small amounts in various animal products, such as beef, pork, lamb, and the butterfat in butter and milk.
    - Hydrogenated fats are chemically altered fats. Trans-fatty acids are also formed during hydrogenation.
    - Both trans fats and hydrogenated fats raise total blood cholesterol, raise LDL (bad) cholesterol, and lower HDL (good) cholesterol.

- Trans-fatty acids (hydrogenated fats) are found in fast food, fried foods, processed foods, and many man-made food products (see Junk Food, #14).
- The long-term health effects of trans-fatty acids are unknown, but they do contribute to an increase in body fat and water retention.

- MY DIVA DIET wants you to know that not all fats are bad. Some are good, some marginal, some unhealthy. You should eliminate bad fats, eat moderate ones sparingly, and include good fats in your diet.
- A fat-free diet is not recommended.

✳ Total Daily Fat Intake Rules

- In the Diva Reduction Phase, eat no more than 30 grams of good fat per day.
  - Use your 30 grams per day wisely because they add up quickly.
- In the Diva Maintenance Phase, healthy fat grams can increase somewhat.
- To help you further in choosing good fats, see Quality Fat Intake (#21).

16. Total daily sugar intake (grams)

Overconsumption of sugar is a rapidly growing problem in America today. The Center for Science in the Public Interest notes that we eat 20% more sugar now than in 1986. The average American eats twenty teaspoons of added sugar a day, aside from natural forms of sugar like lactose in milk and fructose in fruit. With so much sugar being consumed, it's no wonder we face growing problems with obesity, diabetes, gout, and other health issues.

✳ Notes

- One level teaspoon of table sugar contains 15 empty calories, which means that these calories have little, if any, nutritional value.
- Beyond the sugar we add to our coffee or tea, we consume sugar in a myriad of packaged foods where its content is disguised by other names, like "high fructose corn syrup", which can cause fat gain and health problems.
  - Read the ingredients panel on just some of the hundreds of cereals currently on the market today.
    - Then compare Frosted Flakes and Trix (each of which has between 11 and 13 grams of sugar per cup) to Kashi and Erewhon cereals (each of which has less than one gram) and to Arrowhead Mills and Ancient Quinoa (each of which has zero sugar grams).

- Just because you don't use table sugar or eat high-sugar cereals doesn't mean you are avoiding sugar in your diet. Just read the labels on other packaged, man-made food products.
  - Be aware of other sources of sugar, like molasses, syrup, jams, etc.

* Total Daily Sugar Intake Rules
- Avoid eating or adding table sugar to your food.
- Since there is plenty of sugar occurring naturally in some foods (e.g. dairy products, fruits, vegetables), try to keep your extra sugar intake to no more than 50 grams per day.
  - Be very selective in your extra sugar sources.
    - Use honey (1 Tbsp. = 17 g) or agave nectar (1 Tbsp. = 8.2 g).
- Begin to read labels on packaged foods—you will be truly amazed at how many products contain sugar and/or sugar derivatives.
- Train your taste buds to start enjoying the natural tastes of whole food and liquids, and you will reap the rewards of a leaner body, better health, and a more vibrant look. And, you will avoid many potential health issues.

* FYI's
- Other sweeteners for MY DIVA DIET (sugar grams):
  - No-sugar-added applesauce: 1/2 cup = 11 grams
  - 100% fruit spread: 1 Tbsp. = 9 grams
- Fruit gives you sweetness and nutrition at the same time—try dried fruit with no additives (three figs = 20 grams).
  - Be carefull of eating too much dried fruit—it is a concentrated source of sugar and high in calories.

* Special Notes on Chocolate
- Plain dark chocolate provides some health benefits:
  - It contains traces of iron, calcium, and potassium, and vitamins A, B1, C, D, and E.
  - It is also one of the highest natural sources of magnesium.
- Keep in mind that other ingredients—primarily sugar—are added to chocolate.

* Chocolate Rules
- Eating dark chocolate may be okay from time to time, but it should be as pure as possible.
- Always choose dark chocolate over milk chocolate or white chocolate.
- Dark chocolate is a smart diet cheat—just don't eat a one-pound bar.

* FYI's
- On average, one ounce of dark chocolate = 150 calories, 10 grams of fat, and 12.6 grams of sugar.
- Plain dark chocolate usually has around four ingredients: about 71% cocoa solids, 29% sugar, vegetable lecithin, and vanilla.

17. Sugar substitutes (artificial sweeteners)

Artificial sweeteners are chemicals that offer the sweet flavor of sugar without the calories. There is much debate on their safety and MY DIVA DIET does not recommend them.

* Notes
- The long-term harmful effects of some artificial sweeteners are documented. However, as new ones come on the market, their effects will remain unknown until the harm is already done.
  - According to some researchers, nutritionists, and diabetes experts, artificial sweeteners may have carcinogenic properties and be linked to increased risk of tumors, seizure disorders, chronic headaches, and hyperactivity in children.

* Sugar Substitutes Rule
- To become genuinely healthy & fit you should avoid unnecessary sugar and artificial sweeteners while developing a taste for foods and liquids in their natural forms.

18. Total daily sodium intake (milligrams)

Sodium is a mineral that helps our nerves and muscles function properly, aids in the absorption of major nutrients, and helps maintain an adequate water and mineral balance. However, the typical American diet includes three to five times more sodium than we need.

An important side note: To add to the problem of sodium overconsumption, our inadequate intake of other important minerals—like calcium, magnesium, potassium, and others—not only affects our overall health & fitness, but can create a harmful imbalance in electrolytes. Our bodies require a proper electrolyte balance to regulate important functions like nerve reactions and muscle functions.

✱ Notes

- Sodium becomes a problem when we consume it in excess. We add table salt to our meals and recipes; eat processed, canned, packaged, and fast food; and eat out frequently at non-health-food restaurants where we don't know what kind of seasoning the chef is using.
  - Excessive sodium can cause fluid retention in blood vessels, making our hearts work harder and resulting in high blood pressure.
  - Excessive sodium can make us look and feel bloated by causing us to retain water subcutaneously (i.e., under our skin) rather than in our muscles.

✱ Total Daily Sodium Intake Rules

- MY DIVA DIET recommends that you consume approximately one milligram of sodium per calorie (or slightly over or under). So, if you are eating 1,300 calories per day, you should consume only about 1,300 milligrams of sodium per day (if you are exercising and sweating, you can consume more sodium—just make sure it comes from natural sources).
- MY DIVA DIET recommends not only that you decrease sodium intake by choosing healthy foods, but that you increase your intake of potassium and other important minerals.
- Read labels to look for total sodium content and sodium derivatives like sodium nitrite, sorbate, sulfite, etc.—there are too many to list here and some of them are actually harmful.
  - It is better to skip most processed, packaged, canned, frozen, and man-made foods entirely, as they are packed with sodium and sodium derivatives.
- Consume sodium the natural way by drinking water and eating wholesome foods in their natural state.
- Cook without salt, using fruits, vegetables, herbs, and spices to enhance your dishes.
- Remove the salt shaker from your table and train your taste buds to enjoy the natural flavors of real foods—use pepper instead!

- If you must use salt, use kosher salt or sea salt and use it sparingly.

✱ FYI's
- We at MY DIVA DIET always hear, "I don't use salt on my food, so I don't get sodium in my diet." Just in case you think you aren't consuming much sodium, be aware that many non-junk foods contain sodium. And, as mentioned earlier, restaurant dining doesn't give you control over the salt used in the meals you order—unless you ask.
- Because sodium is an important nutrient, going sodium-free is not the answer either. The following table presents some foods that contain sodium naturally:

FOOD CHART

Food	Quantity	Sodium (mg)
Meats and poultry	3 oz.	50 to 70
Fish	3 oz.	40 to 70
Eggs	1 (whole)	65
Dairy		
Milk	8 oz.	100 to 125
Cheese	1 oz.	90 to 100
Yogurt	1 cup	100 to 175
Vegetables	1/2 to 1 cup	0 to 151
Potato	1	16

19. Quality protein intake

Proteins are the primary building blocks of muscles, tendons, ligaments, organs, and glands. Adequate protein is mandatory for growth and development in children and adolescents and for optimum wellness in children and adults.

- MY DIVA DIET recommends that high-quality protein account for approximately 35% of your daily calories in the Diva Reduction Phase and 20 to 35% in the Diva Maintenance Phase.

❋ Notes
- There are bad and good protein choices, and choosing quality proteins will help you live a healthy & fit life. Examples of good-quality protein sources are:
  - Organic, cage-free chicken, turkey, and eggs
  - Antibiotic-free, hormone-free meat from grass-fed, free-range livestock
  - Wild, mercury-free fish
  - Organic dairy and dairy products
  - Plant sources such as organic legumes, nuts, and seeds
- Kosher ("fit to eat") meats and foods are produced as even healthier, higher-quality sources of protein.
  - No hormones or antibiotics are used in kosher meats and foods.
  - The kosher method of slaughtering livestock is now being recognized as the most humane.
  - Kosher meat has been proven to be healthier and better-tasting than non-kosher meat.
- Poor-quality proteins come from these sources:
  - Caged chickens fed unnatural poor-quality feed and not allowed to roam freely
  - Overcrowded livestock injected with antibiotics and hormones
  - Livestock fed with unnatural feed
  - Farm-raised fish fed unnatural land-based diets that contain little or no omega-3 fatty acids and are often contaminated with PCB and mercury
- Whatever the quality of our protein sources, we can ruin them by overcooking
- Cooking at very high heat may activate cancer-causing agents in red meat, poultry, and fish.

❋ Quality Protein Intake Rules
- Not enough protein is detrimental to your health and ability to get lean, but too much protein can be toxic.
  - In the Diva Reduction Phase MY DIVA DIET recommends approximately 100 to 120 grams of protein each day.
  - In the Diva Maintenance Phase you can go lower than this. Higher would not be a good idea unless you have 150 pounds of lean body mass and/or you are an athlete.

- Animal protein: Stay away from heavily processed animal products and foods, meats injected with hormones and antibiotics, and farm-raised fish.
- Dairy protein: Choose low-fat or non-fat organic dairy and dairy products (rice milk is a good alternative to dairy milk).
- Plant protein (legumes, nuts, and seeds): This is a great way to get your protein and some fiber at the same time and a good way to replace dairy—make sure your choices are pure, and that any added ingredients are few and healthy.
  - Try germinating and/or sprouting your own beans, nuts, and seeds for a pure and extremely nutritious food.
  - Soybeans (edamame) are healthful and delicious, as are soy products like soy milk, soy yogurt, soy butter, soy cheese, and tofu.
  - Hummus (made from chickpeas) is another good source of plant protein.
  - Make sure nuts and seeds are raw and not coated with sugar or salt.
- The following is a quick-glance chart to help you choose wholesome animal protein:

Paw Animal Protein Guide

Animal Protein*	Best Choice	Note
Eggs	Egg whites (occasional whole eggs)	Buy cage-free, organic, veg fed
Poultry	Lean white meat	Buy skinless or remove skin
Beef	Lean kosher beef (trim fat, eat rarely)	Look for the kosher triangle ⚠K
Seafood ✱	Clean, cooked fish	Buy fresh, wild fish with fins and scales

*Note: Choose kosher for all animal protein

✱ Avoid swordfish, sturgeon, shark, flatfish, catfish, sculpins, and monkfish.
✱ Avoid mollusks (clams, mussels, oysters, scallops).
✱ Avoid crustaceans (crabs, lobster, shrimp, prawns, crayfish).

See our full list of animal protein choices in the Diva Reduction Good Food Choices At-a-Glance (PART SIX).

* Special Notes on Seafood
- For years nutritionists have known that seafood is a top-quality source of protein, containing all nine essential amino acids and enabling us to meet our daily protein needs.
- Seafood has other health benefits:
  - It is highly digestible.
  - It is also considered an excellent source of B complex, calcium, and other minerals.
  - It is naturally low in sodium, low in calories, and low in saturated fat.
- The omega-3 fatty acids found in some seafood are important for a healthy diet.
  - Omega-3 fatty acids offer a variety of health benefits, including but not limited to reducing inflammation throughout the body, keeping blood from clotting excessively, lowering lipids in the bloodstream, helping prevent cancer cell growth, and helping reduce the risk of obesity.
  - Certain kinds of seafood are excellent sources of omega-3 fatty acids, including salmon, sardines, and tuna.
  - Halibut and snapper have high amounts of omega-3 fatty acids, as does other seafood.
  - It is difficult to get your omega-3 fatty acids without consuming seafood.
    - If you don't like seafood or are a vegetarian, consider supplementing with fish oil or getting omega-3 from leafy green vegetables, nuts, seeds, hummus, some oils, and eggs.

* Special Notes on Processed Meats and Meat Products
- While lunch meats are better than sausages, hot dogs, and other meat products, they are still processed. The quality of the meat used is sometimes questionable, and they contain many ingredients (including sugar) and are very high in salt, nitrites, starch, dextrose, fat, and other questionable ingredients.
  - Most pre-sliced, packaged deli lunch meats:
    - Are taken from a single animal part
    - Are minimally processed
    - Contain low levels of fat and high levels of protein
  - Most sausage and loaf lunch meats:
    - Contain multiple parts of an animal

- Are highly processed
- Contain high quantities of fat and sodium
- Turkey and chicken breast lunch meats are better and leaner than salami, bologna, ham, and roast beef.
- Meat by-products:
  - Are full of many harmful ingredients and items you might not expect (e.g. crushed animal bones, pork brains, and more)
  - Contain 1200% of recommended daily cholesterol

✱ Special Notes on Hot Dogs, Veggie and Tofu Dogs, and Kosher Dogs
- Hot dogs mostly are full of mechanically separated meats and high levels of fat, sodium, and nitrites. Some of the better ones contain higher-grade meats, less sodium, and fewer preservatives.
  - Traditional hot dogs are made of beef, pork, or a combination of the two.
  - Turkey and chicken hot dogs also are available.
  - Veggie and tofu dogs are available but are not particularly wholesome.
    - Smart Dogs contain water, soy protein isolate, wheat gluten, evaporated cane sugar, salt, yeast extract, soy sauce (water, soybeans, wheat, salt), granulated garlic, carrageenan, spice extract, natural flavors (from vegetable sources), vegetable gum, natural smoke flavor, potassium chloride, and tomato pulp.
    - Tofu Pups are made from water soy protein isolate, soy oil, organic spray dried tofu (organic dehulled soybeans, calcium sulfate), 2% natural flavors from vegetable sources (beet powder, yeast extract, sunflower oil, natural smoke flavor, salt, paprika oleorsin, vegetable gums, and tomato pulp), no nitrites, and no MSG.
  - Kosher dogs use the highest quality meat and contain minimal artificial flavors, colors, fillers, or by-products.
    - Hebrew National hot dogs contain about nine ingredients (beef, water, salt, spices, hydrolyzed soy protein, garlic powder, sodium erythorbate, sodium nitrite, and flavorings). (Hebrew National at www.hebrewnational.com).

✱ Special Notes on Beef and Turkey Jerky and Smoked Fish
- Jerky is created by marinating and cutting lean meat into thin strips and then drying it under low heat or in the sun. The meat is preserved, so it is high in sodium and other preservatives.
  - Processed jerky is actually a meat paste, so it is less nutritious.

- Organic jerky usually contains no preservatives, no added MSG, no nitrites, no erythorbate, no artificial ingredients, and is only minimally processed.
  - It usually has a shorter shelf life.
  - It also has higher amounts of protein and less fat and sodium.
    - One serving of Jerky Direct (a few slices) = 60 calories, 11 grams of protein, 6 grams of carbs, and 0 grams of fat. It contains 270 milligrams of sodium and 5 grams of sugar. Ingredients include turkey, sugar, water, soy sauce (water, wheat, soybeans, salt), apple cider vinegar, salt, flavorings, paprika, natural smoke flavorings, and caramel color. (www.jerkydirect.com).
- Smoked fish also includes many ingredients, preservatives, and additives, and consists of fish of varying quality.
- Kosher smoked fish contains farm-raised Atlantic salmon, astaxanthin and/or canthaxanthin as added color, salt, sugar, sodium nitrite, and oakwood smoke. (www.aaronsgourmet.com).

* Rules on Processed Meats and Other Meat Products

- Because of the high amounts of preservatives and additives, as well as factory processing, MY DIVA DIET does not recommend processed meats and meat products as part of your daily diet, especially in the Diva Reduction Phase.
  - Ham, bologna, pastrami, and salami should not be consumed.
  - Sausage and hot dogs (including veggie dogs) are not recommended.
- The exceptions to this general rule include:
  - Occasional lunch meat like chicken and turkey breast cuts, or roast beef from your local deli.
  - Boar's Head deli meats (www.boarshead.com)—they and similar high-quality deli meats contain no by-products, gluten, trans fats, cereals, fillers, artificial flavors, or colors.
  - Having a kosher hot dog or veggie dog may be okay on occasion if the ingredients are pure.
  - Occasional dried meat or smoked fish is okay. Just note that these are similar to dried fruit—higher in calories and sodium for a smaller portion.

20. Quality carbohydrate intake

Carbohydrates are the most desirable fuel source, supplying our bodies with the energy we need for daily living. Eating the proper kind of carbohydrates will keep us from getting fat and developing possible health problems like diabetes and coronary heart disease.

- MY DIVA DIET recommends that high-quality carbohydrates account for approximately 45% of your daily calories in the Diva Reduction Phase and 45% to 65% in the Diva Maintenance Phase.

* Notes
- There are two categories of carbohydrates: complex and simple.
  - Good carbohydrates are the complex ones, like fruit and vegetables, whole grains and grain foods, and legumes.
    - Potatoes and yams are excellent choices for healthy complex carbohydrates.
  - Poor-quality carbohydrates are the simple ones, like sugar, processed foods, soft drinks, snacks like cookies and chips, and alcohol.
    - Most simple carbohydrates are highly refined, contain huge amounts of calories, contribute no nutritional value or fiber, and leave you feeling hungry.

* The Carb Defense
- Ever since the "no-carb" craze, carbohydrates have gotten a bad rap—particularly grains. Many of us know the health benefits of consuming fruits and vegetables but are unaware of the benefits derived from grains.
  - Fruits and vegetables not only provide many vitamins, minerals, and fiber, but their attractive rainbow colors indicate natural plant pigments that contain specific important nutrients and help prevent certain types of cancers and other diseases.
  - Whole grains give us the sustained energy we need each day and also provide:
    - Fiber, which helps reduce blood cholesterol, may lower the risk of heart disease, reduces constipation and diverticulosis, and helps you feel full (so you eat fewer calories).
    - Folic acid and other B vitamins, which play a key role in metabolism, help the body release energy from protein, fat, and carbohydrates; and are essential for a healthy nervous system.
    - Several minerals that are directly related to the proper function of our bodies and immune system.
    - Antioxidants and phytoestrogens, which are helpful in preventing some forms of cancer, fighting off menopausal symptoms, and decreasing the risk of some chronic diseases.

- Whole grains like wheat and barley have young sprouts known as cereal grasses that contain antioxidant enzymes, trace minerals, chlorophyll, and high-quality vegetable proteins that create a powerful tool for good health—e.g. wheat grass.
- Since fruits, vegetables, and grains are crucial for health and actually can help with weight loss, think again before you eliminate them from your diet. Case closed!

✱ Quality Carbohydrate Intake Rule
- Unlike other diet programs, MY DIVA DIET doesn't want you to avoid carbohydrates. We just want you to clean them up and control the amount you consume.
- 200 grams or less of carbohydrates seem to be the best amount to consume each day for most women to lose fat, stay healthy, and be able to function.
  - In the Diva Reduction Phase (based on 1,300 calories per day) MY DIVA DIET recommends about 130 to 150 grams. Under 100 grams per day is just not safe—you will not get leaner quicker, nor will you maintain your results.
  - In the Diva Maintenance Phase, you can go higher in carbohydrates (how high depends on many variables).
  - If you are exercising, have a high metabolism, or for other reasons listed in our Daily caloric intake, #9), a higher carbohydrate intake is warranted.
- Avoid simple carbohydrates like table sugar, junk food, cookies, donuts, etc., as these are not only unhealthy but add unwanted fat pounds to your body.
  - The only high-sugar carbohydrates that may be okay in moderation are honey, agave nectar, natural fruit spreads, applesauce, and some dried fruits with no additives.
- Choose your carbohydrates from natural, fresh, organic fruits and vegetables, whole grains, and legumes.
- Choose a variety of fruits and vegetables to ensure that you get every benefit nature has to offer. Look for these colors: red, orange, yellow, green, blue/purple, and white.
- Be very selective when choosing grain products and use the following Paw Guide:

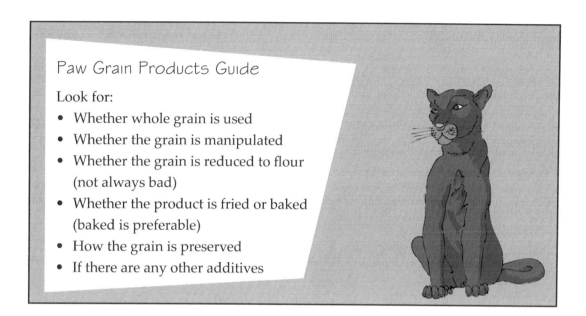

Paw Grain Products Guide

Look for:
- Whether whole grain is used
- Whether the grain is manipulated
- Whether the grain is reduced to flour (not always bad)
- Whether the product is fried or baked (baked is preferable)
- How the grain is preserved
- If there are any other additives

21. Quality fat intake

In fats, just as with proteins and carbohydrates, there are good, marginal, and bad choices. Our bodies need good-quality fats because they help with nutrient absorption, nerve transmissions, and cell membrane integrity. When we consume marginal fats in excess and bad fats regularly, they take their toll with weight gain, heart disease, certain types of cancer, and an array of other health issues.

- MY DIVA DIET recommends that high-quality fats account for approximately 20% of your daily calories in the Diva Reduction Phase and 20 to 30% in the Diva Maintenance Phase.
  - Extra-lean Divas can go as low as 15% fat.

* Notes
- As noted earlier (Total daily fat intake, #15), some fats are good, some marginal, and some bad.
  - Good fats are monounsaturated and polyunsaturated fats, which can be found in salmon and other seafood, nuts and seeds, and olive oil, as well as in canola, soy, soybean, safflower, and sunflower oils.
  - Medium-grade fats (okay in moderation) include saturated fats and foods containing cholesterol (meat, dairy, eggs, some seafood, and coconut and palm oils).

- Bad fat choices are those products that contain trans fats and hydrogenated fats (mainly found in some man-made food products, especially fast foods, fried foods, packaged snacks, vegetable shortening, hard-stick margarine, etc.).

✱ Quality Fat Intake Rules
- Quality of fats is always of utmost importance.
  - In the Diva Reduction Phase, keep your good fats to 30 grams per day or less.
  - In the Diva Maintenance Phase, you can increase them somewhat.
- Eliminate bad fats from your diet first, eat moderate ones sparingly, and incorporate good fats into your diet. This approach will help you lose fat and be much healthier.

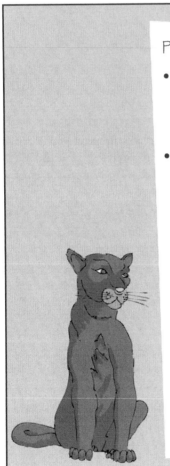

Paw 'Trim the Fat' Guide
- Add good fats to your diet by:
  - Eating wholesome foods in their natural forms (especially fish, nuts, seeds, avocados, and olive oil)
- Cut bad fats from your diet by:
  - Choosing lean cuts of beef and poultry
  - Trimming skin and visible fat from meats
  - Avoiding poultry skin
  - Switching to egg whites
  - Choosing low-fat to no-fat dairy products
  - Watching the amount of cheese and butter you eat
  - Being cautious of dressings, sauces, and dips
  - Watching for saturated fats and cholesterol in natural and packaged foods
  - Reading labels to avoid trans fats and hydrogenated oils
  - Avoiding most packaged, processed foods
  - Avoiding fried and fast foods

22. Total daily dairy intake

Although Americans consume some milk and milk products from sheep and goats, the American diet derives most of its dairy products from cattle. We at MY DIVA DIET love cows and know that dairy is big business, but there are mixed reviews from nutritionists, fitness professionals, and even those in the medical field about the benefits of cattle dairy products, ranging from the belief that they are harmful to the conviction that they are a great food source. MY DIVA DIET takes the middle ground and finds dairy and dairy products acceptable as long as they are clean and pure and are not consumed in excess.

* Notes
- We tend to drink too much dairy (milk) and eat too many foods and products that contain dairy, and there are drawbacks to this habit.
  - The lactose that is found in milk (and all dairy products) is a form of naturally occurring sugar, but many dairy products contain added sugar (for example, some yogurts = 36 grams of carbohydrates, and 31 of them are from sugar).
  - Dairy and dairy products do have some protein, but they are high in fat unless you get low- or non-fat types (the two exceptions are cottage cheese and some yogurts).
  - Unless you use organic dairy and dairy products, you risk the possibility of consuming a product from a cow that was injected with hormones and antibiotics. Also, consider the cow's feed (which affects its milk) as well as its health, treatment, and living conditions.
  - The big push for milk is because of the calcium it contains, but you can select other healthy foods that are good sources of calcium.
    - In one cup of beet greens, broccoli, chicory, Chinese cabbage, collard greens, kale, rhubarb, or spinach you can get anywhere from 10% to 35% of the RDA (recommended daily allowance) of calcium without the fat, sugar, or sodium.
      - These foods also provide other important vitamins, minerals, and fiber.
    - You can also get calcium from sardines and salmon, tofu, soy or rice milk, soybeans, nuts and seeds, and other leafy green vegetables.

* Total Daily Dairy Intake Rules

- Dairy and dairy products are okay but are not the total answer to your mineral requirements and can add unhealthy calories to your diet (unless you are extremely careful with your choices). Your best bet is to keep dairy and dairy product consumption down to one to two times per day (or less if you can).
  - Less dairy (except for yogurt) is best when you are trying to lose weight, but this also holds true for maintenance and overall health.
- Choose low-fat or non-fat organic milk & cottage cheese and low- or non-fat, no-sugar-added yogurts.
  - Cottage cheese is a great way to get protein into your diet.
  - Yogurt is a good source of acidophilus—a beneficial bacteria that helps prevent the growth of harmful bacteria in the body (gastrointestinal tract).
    - Choose yogurt and cottage cheese that contain live active cultures.
- Because of its high fat content, cheese should be consumed in small amounts.
  - In the Diva Reduction Phase, Parmesan, Romano, feta, skim mozzarella, and string cheese are acceptable because a small amount goes a long way.
  - In the Diva Maintenance Phase, you can add other kinds of cheese in small amounts.
- Other commonly used dairy products are butter and cream. These are high in fat and should be used sparingly.
- For those of you who are lactose-intolerant (unable to absorb the natural sugar in dairy) or who don't really care for dairy, rice or soy milk and other soy and rice products are good choices.
- Be aware that dairy is used as an ingredient in many other foods, so you need to monitor this aspect as well.
- Try goat's milk—e.g. popular alternative to cow's milk.

* FYI

The following is some nutritional information on a variety of dairy products:

FOOD CHART

Product	Protein (g)	Carbs (g)	Fat (g)	Calcium (% RDA)	Sodium (mg)	Potassium (mg)	B12 (% RDA)
Milk (1 cup low fat)	8	11.7	2.6	38%	123	380.9	45%
Cheddar cheese (1 oz.)	7	.4	9.3	25%	174	28	12%
Cottage cheese (1/2 cup low fat)	14	3.1	1.2	9%	459	108	36%
Yogurt (1 cup low fat)	11.9	16	3.5	52%	159	530.7	64%
Vanilla ice cream (1/2 cup)	2.1	16	11.9	9%	54	186	14%

* Special Notes on Pasteurized vs. Raw Milk
- Whether pasteurized or raw milk is better for you is an area of much debate.
  - Pasteurized milk is heated at high temperatures to destroy undesirable bacteria. Some health professionals claim that the way milk is processed today not only destroys bad bacteria but can also destroy enzymes, diminish vitamin content, denature milk proteins, alter some B vitamins, kill beneficial bacteria, and promote pathogens. They also claim it is associated with allergies, increased tooth decay, colic in infants, and much more.
  - The belief that raw milk is healthier is disputed by public health officials, who claim that raw milk may harbor a host of food-borne disease-causing organisms (pathogens) such as the bacteria carnpylobacter, escheria, listeria, salmonella, yersnia, and brucella.
- While MY DIVA DIET's philosophy is always to choose fresh foods in their natural state over processed or genetically modified foods, dairy is a difficult call.
  - The FDA and dairy farmers tend to have different agendas.
  - You may be safer with pasteurized milk because raw milk may come from cows that aren't kept healthy and happy.

- If you can do some research and find a dairy company you trust, you may want to go with raw milk.

23. Clean calories (reading labels/things to look for)
   - Preservatives and additives
   - Flavoring agents, coloring agents, sweeteners (artificial and natural), emulsifiers, texturizers, stabilizers, etc.
   - Chemicals and other fake foods
   - Hidden fats (hydrogenated vegetable oils and other unneeded and unhealthy fats)
   - Hidden sugars (maltodextrin, corn syrup, high fructose corn syrup, etc.)
   - Hidden sodium (salt, MSG, sodium benzoate, sodium nitrate, ferrous sulfate, etc.)
   - Hidden flour (white flour, baking powder, starch, dextrin, etc.)

Always know what you are eating and what the ingredients in your food are—or at least have a good idea (do your own research). This major adjustment to old eating habits will guarantee weight loss, improved health, and longer life.

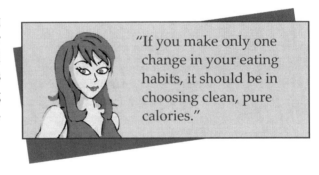

"If you make only one change in your eating habits, it should be in choosing clean, pure calories."

* Notes
- Clean and pure calories are very important in MY DIVA DIET (in both Phase One and Two) because health should be the number one goal in any weight-loss program. In fact, if you are healthy you will find it much easier to lose weight.
- Cleaning up your calories is more important than decreasing your intake, and the best way to do it is to select natural and fresh foods over packaged, processed, man-made foods.
- Some diets are based on eating a great many unclean calories that help you lose a few pounds but place you at risk for health predicaments like fibromyalgia, headaches, heart disease, diabetes, cancer, and others.

* Clean Calories Rule
- There are two main rules in this category:
  - Become informed about food additives and preservatives.
  - Read labels, read labels, read labels!

Paw Ingredients Label Guide

Number of Ingredients	Signals
1	Ideal
3	Excellent
5	Probably OK
6-9	May need further analysis
10-19	Could be a problem
20-29	Caution
30 +	Stay away!

* FYI's
- Ingredients for a given product are listed by weight, in descending order.
- Some preservatives are okay, but not when there are more preservatives than the natural food it is supposed to be made of.
  - Some preservatives are actively harmful—you should do your own research to learn more about food additives.
- Avoid products containing too many additives like colorings, fillers, flavor enhancers, etc.
- Watch for hidden calories, fats, sugar, sodium, and flour.
- Avoid products with unfamiliar ingredients—find out what they are!

24. Purity of calories
  - Natural foods vs. processed
  - Fresh foods vs. man-manipulated
  - Organic vs. non-organic
  - Kosher vs. non-kosher

Fresh foods in their natural states are best in all cases, and organic and kosher are best where applicable and whenever possible.

129

* Notes
- If foods are not marked as organic or kosher, MY DIVA DIET believes that they are either not safe or only partially safe to eat, for reasons noted earlier and listed here.
  - Most animals raised for food (poultry, cattle, etc.) are injected with hormones and antibiotics and sometimes kept in despicable living conditions and slaughtered in a manner that is not only barbaric, but makes our meats toxic.
  - Most farm-raised fish have an imbalance of omega-3 and omega-6 fatty acids. They are less healthy due to being out of their natural environment (the ocean —fresh water).
  - Most commercial fruits and vegetables are contaminated with pesticides meant to kill unwanted bugs. Are pesticides meant for human consumption?
  - Most commercial fruits and vegetables are grown in substandard soil and are picked too early and sold too late, thus lacking some important nutrients and the great taste these foods naturally offer.
  - Designer foods—genetically engineered foods that are man-manipulated—are another concern because their long-term effects remain unknown.
  - Frozen, packaged, and canned foods will add unwanted weight to your body and may cause many long-term health problems.
    - These foods were created for increased shelf life, but because of this they are full of sodium, sugar, and fats and their derivatives, as well as chemicals and fillers.
    - Some of these foods are manipulated to change their taste, thus diminishing their true flavors and stripping them of their nutrients.
  - Restaurant eating contributes to the obesity problem because of the pervasive use of sugar, salt, fats, flour, and other ingredients not conducive to health & fitness. You also lack control in ensuring that your food is natural, fresh, organic, and kosher.

* Special Notes on Organic Foods
- Organic foods keep you from consuming harmful pesticides, hormones, and antibiotics.
- Organic foods are also much higher in antioxidants, provide better nutritional value, contribute to overall health, and taste better.

* Special Notes on Kosher Meats

- Animals raised for kosher meats lead happier, healthier lives and are slaughtered in a more humane manner, resulting in healthier meats.
  - Happier lives for animals means better health and thus a higher-quality meat.
  - The lack of stress and fear at slaughter means no adrenaline is released into the meat, affecting its quality.
- Because of its higher quality, kosher meat also tastes much better.
- Eating kosher meats will also make our consciences more fit.

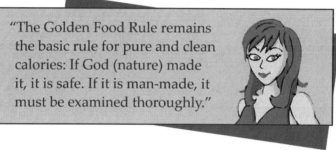

"The Golden Food Rule remains the basic rule for pure and clean calories: If God (nature) made it, it is safe. If it is man-made, it must be examined thoroughly."

* Purity of Calories Rules

- Keep your calories clean and pure—natural and fresh.
- Try to eat organic and kosher foods as much as possible.
  - Only about 15% of man-manipulated foods are safe.
  - Eliminate most—and in some cases all—processed, packaged, canned, and fast food because fresh live food is what our bodies need to be healthy & fit.
    - There are some canned and frozen foods that are safe, but you should be extremely selective in your choice: Try canned plain legumes; frozen peas, corn, fruits, and treats; some canned tuna; olives; and organic soups (there are other exceptions not listed—just read the labels).

- For a simple summary of this information, use the following Paw Food Guide (first presented in PART ONE):

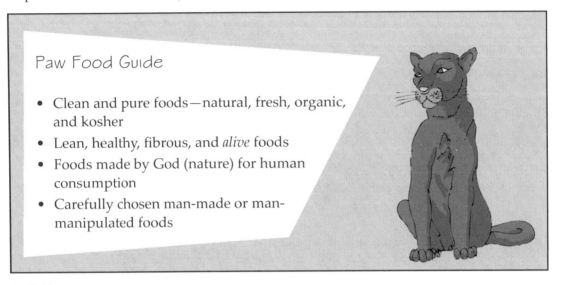

Paw Food Guide

- Clean and pure foods—natural, fresh, organic, and kosher
- Lean, healthy, fibrous, and *alive* foods
- Foods made by God (nature) for human consumption
- Carefully chosen man-made or man-manipulated foods

* FYI's
  - Food for Life rice and sprouted corn tortillas
  - Kashi 7 Grain Cereal Puffs
  - Erewhon Crispy Brown Rice Cereal Puffs
  - Back to Nature rice thins
  - Real Foods corn thins
  - Lundberg rice cakes
  - Health Seed spelt or rye bread
  - Annie's Natural low-fat dressing
  - Sorrell Ridge 100% fruit spread
  - Trader Joe's and Laura Scudders nut butter
  - Barbara's Bakery wheat-free fig bars
  - 100% Natural Fruit Stix fruit bars
- The following chart contains only a few of some common frozen-food entrees that are considered healthy (and labeled that way). We won't address canned foods and other packaged foods, they would take up our entire book. MY DIVA DIET wants you to read and compare the labels on these and other products before you choose any packaged, processed, or man-made food products.

FOOD CHART

Entrée	Calories	Protein (g)	Carbs (g)	Fat (g)	Sugar	Sodium (mg)	Fiber	Ingredients
Amy's Bowls Brown Rice and Vegetables	260	9	36	9	7	550	5	About 30 All organic/ No trans fats, MSG, or preservatives
South Beach Diet Caprese Chicken w/Broccoli	260	33	12	7	4	710	4	About 50
Smart Ones Chicken Fettuccini	340	23	47	6	3	680	4	About 50+
Lean Cuisine Lemongrass Chicken	240	17	30	6	4	600	4	About 55
Kashi Sweet and Sour Chicken	320	18	55	3.5	25	380	6	About 60
Lean Cuisine Panini	280	21	32	8	3	690	5	MANY
Lean Pockets (1)	290	11	45	7	5	500	5	MANY
Healthy Choice Roasted Chicken	290	16	39	7	7	600	10	MANY
Smart Ones 3-Cheese Macaroni	300	14	48	6	3	570	3	MANY
Stouffer's Rigatoni w/Roasted Chicken	390	19	44	15	2	820	3	MANY

25. White flour intake (bread, cereals, crackers, noodles, pasta, pastries, tortillas, etc.)

White flour encompasses a big part of the American diet. It is included not only in the previous food chart but in many others like gravy, dips, and condiments. A diet of refined foods can leave many women malnourished, constipated, and vulnerable to chronic illnesses. We eat a great deal of white flour—and then wonder why we are sick.

* Notes
- Highly processed white flour (enriched wheat flour) is missing the two most important, nutritious, fibrous parts of the seed: the outside bran layer and the germ (embryo).
  - These contain nutrients like fiber, B-complex vitamins (thiamine, riboflavin, niacin, and folate), and iron and trace minerals.
- Phytochemicals (naturally-occurring health-promoting substances found in fruits, vegetables, whole grains, legumes, and nuts) are also lost during the refining process.
- Other ingredients we need to be leery of are the ones we frequently use in our cooking and baking and that are found in many man-made products: breads and baked goods, beer, wine, cereal, waffles, pancakes, pudding, sauces, condiments, etc. Common ingredients found in these products include yeast, starch and starch derivatives like maltodextrin, and baking powder, just to name a few.

* White Flour Intake Rules
- Avoid white flour (enriched wheat flour).
- Select breads and other products made with grains (grain products) that use the whole grain and have the whole grain listed first on the ingredients panel.
- Some of the best grain products are "sprouted" grains which provide better nutrition, enhanced digestion, and less allergic potential. You can find good sprouted products at:
  - Food For Life (www.foodforlife.com)
  - Trader Joe's sprouted breads and other healthy grain products (www.traderjoes.com)
  - Your local health food store

- "Stone ground" grains are also wholesome, and are usually coarser and have the germ intact. The bran portion may or may not be included.
- Be sure to check the ingredients in man-made food products for white flour and other baking ingredients, which should be avoided.
- Be extremely cautious with pancakes, waffles, muffins, tortillas, etc., even if they are labeled healthy.

✻ FYI's and Other Flour Rules
- Wheat is not the only grain used to make flour. Others include amaranth, arrowroot, barley, buckwheat, corn, flaxseed, kamut, oats, quinoa, rice, rye, soy, spelt, teff, and triticale.
- Vegetable and nut flours are also available, including bean flour, chickpea flour, chestnut flour, peasemeal (pea flour), potato flour, sweet potato flour, and almond and hazelnut flours.
- Flour and products made with flour other than wheat or white are okay to eat providing the other ingredients are clean and pure.

26. Total daily fiber intake (grams)
Proper intake of fiber is a major area of neglect in the American diet. We simply don't eat enough fiber, which is very important in preventing and relieving constipation, lowering risk of diabetes and heart disease, fighting colon and intestinal problems, and helping eliminate toxins from our bodies.

✻ Notes
- Eating foods high in fiber helps lower body fat and provides health benefits.
  - Fiber helps you feel full so you won't overeat.
  - Most fibrous foods are low-glycemic, which keeps our blood glucose level steady, enabling our body to burn calories more efficiently—not store them as fat.
  - We can also combine a high-fiber food with a food that is higher on the glycemic index, which will help alleviate a spike in our blood glucose level.
  - Regular bowel movements are not only indicative of good health, but the quicker the transit time, the less likelihood your food will make you sick and fat.
- Our eating habits inhibit our daily fiber intake.
  - We eat too many packaged, processed, and man-made foods. Once you take a food out of its natural state, you have most likely removed the fiber, even in vegetables.

- We don't eat enough vegetables, but when we do, we tend to overcook them, removing many of their nutrients and fiber.
- We fail to eat enough fresh fruits, whole grains, legumes, nuts, and seeds.

* Total Daily Fiber Intake Rules
- Ensure that you are eating at least 25 to 35 grams of fiber each day, spread throughout the day, mainly from fresh fruits and vegetables, whole grains, legumes, nuts, and seeds.
- Think fiber: For each meal you plan or eat, ask yourself, "Where's the fiber?" and count your fiber grams each day.
- Avoid most processed foods, as they will only constipate you and cause other problems.
- Be careful of packaged and man-made foods.

27. Food, sports, energy, and protein bars

The problem with food, sports, energy, and protein bars is that most of them are man-made products with many ingredients. MY DIVA DIET is sure these products were designed with good intentions, but they fail the "real and natural" food test.

* Notes
- There are too many food, sports, energy, and protein bars (alias "food bars") to list here or analyze, and not all of them are created equal. Some are healthier than others, using real ingredients, while others are just glorified candy bars.
- Food bars (including granola bars) are only marginally better for you than candy bars or fast food burgers.
  - Most food bars are high in calories, contain sugar (or high fructose corn syrup), wheat and other flour, fat and fat sources (like hydrogenated oil), salt, milk products, nuts, cocoa and cocoa powder, caffeine and other stimulants, ginseng, and additives and preservatives.
  - Some food bars add vitamins and minerals to increase their value.
  - Some food bars contain fiber and some are gluten-free.

* Food, Sports, Energy, and Protein Bars Rules
- MY DIVA DIET does not recommend food, sports, energy, or protein bars as part of your daily diet—we remind you that you need to get your calories from natural, fresh, and wholesome foods.

- It's okay in an emergency situation to have one of these food bars. Try to choose those with fewer ingredients, higher protein and fiber, and no sugars and low to no flavor enhancers, additives, and preservatives. Again—read the labels!

28. Sauces, salad dressing, dips, and condiment intake

Many Americans don't appreciate real food (e.g. food in its natural form). We not only super-size our meals but also put sauces and condiments on everything.

* Note
- Some sauces, salad dressings, dips and condiments are good to use, such as salsa; marinara sauce; low-sodium, no-wheat soy sauce; olive oil; Balsamic vinegar; low-fat salad dressing; mustard; and horseradish.

* Sauces, Salad Dressing, Dips, and Condiment Rules
- Try to eat your foods plain—it's much better for you.
- If you are going to use sauces, salad dressing, dips, and condiments, use them in moderation, and choose ones that have some nutritional value.
  - Choose items that have minimal calories and ingredients.
- Be extremely selective.
  - Watch out for sauces and dips made at restaurants and those you buy at the grocery store. Most are packed full of fat, flour, sugar, sodium, preservatives, and other harmful ingredients.
  - You can find better-quality products at some health food stores—read labels.

29. Cooking and seasoning (fruits, vegetables, herbs, spices)

Meals do not have to be boring to taste delicious! There are many fruits, vegetables, herbs, and spices that add great flavor—and nutrients—to your favorite dishes and give you a whole new approach to cooking. See our full section on herbs and spices in PART SEVEN and MY DIVA DIET Food Preparation, Cooking, and Meal Planning Guide in PART FIVE to help you prepare healthy & fit meals.

* Notes
- Lemons, pears, tomatoes, chili peppers, garlic, basil, cilantro, and oregano provide added flavor to a variety of dishes.

- Even better news is that fruits, vegetables, herbs, and spices give you added nutrients and fiber without too many calories.
- Once you eliminate unneeded ingredients (like sugar, salt, fat, and flour and seasoning products high in sugar, salt, fat, and flour) in your cooking you will discover the genuine tastes of a variety of foods without the extra calories.
- Using fruits, vegetables, herbs, and spices also means you can use less oil and other fattening and unhealthy products to prepare your meals.

✶ Cooking and Seasoning Rules
- Avoid using table salt, sugar, flour and fats when cooking. Find alternatives in fruits, vegetables, herbs, and spices to eliminate these and add more nutritional value to your meals.
- Avoid microwave cooking, which destroys the enzymes necessary for proper digestion.
- Avoid overcooking, which damages nutrients. *Al dente* and raw foods are best (except for meat, poultry, fish, and eggs, of course).
- There is nothing wrong with eating foods plain—we at MY DIVA DIET do it often.

✶ FYI's on Salt
- A little kosher or sea salt is okay from time to time.
  - Kosher salt is similar to table salt but it contains no additives (like iodine).
  - Sea salt is unrefined salt.
- Avoid table salt, which is composed primarily of refined sodium chloride.

30. Supplement intake (vitamins, minerals, and others)

Vitamins and minerals help us to grow, produce energy, fight disease, repair injured tissue, and maintain normal health. Many of these important nutrients are available in quality, wholesome foods, but supplements are sometimes helpful, especially if we are reducing our calories to lose weight. However, as we adopt better eating habits, our need for supplements should be reduced.

✶ Notes
- In this age of quick fixes, many women try to become healthier or lose fat through prescription medications, diet pills, and supplements like so-called "fat burners", but there is no magic pill to ensure good health, weight loss, or a long life.

- Supplements can be taken to make up for a genuine or possible deficiency in your diet, but they should never replace healthy eating nor are they an answer in and of themselves.

- Relying on supplements can be harmful—you can overdose on some vitamins, minerals, and fat burners if you're not careful.

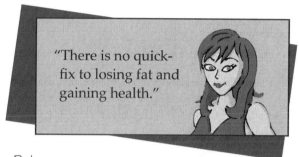

"There is no quick-fix to losing fat and gaining health."

* Supplement Intake Rules

- We at MY DIVA DIET do not encourage excessive pill-taking, but we do realize that it can be difficult for you to get the exact amount of nutrients you need each day in your diet, especially as you attempt to reduce fat.

    - If you are not sure you are getting enough vitamins and minerals from your food, we do recommend that you take a good multivitamin and some additional supplements.

    - If you are under stress, you might consider taking extra vitamin C and B complex since these are water-soluble.

    - Calcium helps maintain bone density and/or offset any bone loss you may experience, especially as you grow older and/or are lacking in exercise.

    - As you age you may need to supplement with other vitamins and minerals.

    - Acidophilus (found in yogurt and cultured milk) is recommended to help balance bacteria in the intestinal tract and counter the potentially damaging effects of antibiotics or other medications.

- Make sure you take your vitamins and minerals with meals rather than on an empty stomach.

* Special supplemental intake circumstances

- Other than daily vitamins and minerals, some natural supplements (when they are warranted) have their purpose: but only after you have carefully evaluated your reason for taking them and the product you about use—consult you doctor and nutritionist and use cautiously. For example: supplements that help with immune function (e.g. Alpha-lipoic acid), joint function (e.g. Glucosamine), nutrient deficiencies (e.g. fish oil and flax seed oil), chemical deficiency (e.g. 5-HTP-amino acid), brain health (e.g. Gingkoba) as well as disease fighting, muscle building, energy producing, and fat loss supplements (like amino acid, enzyme, antioxidant, vitamin, mineral, and herb supplements) – and this is the abbreviated list!

* Special Notes on Natural vs. Synthetic Supplements
- There is much debate over whether natural vitamins are better than synthetic.
  - Natural is always best if you can find the right product and afford it, but it's even better if you eat wholesome foods in their natural states. Then you will get all the vitamins, minerals, antioxidants, amino acids, and enzymes straight from the safest and most pure source possible.
  - Designers, manufacturers, and distributors of supplement brands tend to market their products with exaggerated and sometimes false claims, especially when supplements are labeled as miracle pills. Be cautious, even if they are labeled "natural."

Factor #4: Restrictive and Unbalanced Dieting

31. Restrictive and unbalanced diets
- High-protein, high-fat, no-carbohydrate diets
- Fruit-only diets
- Juice-fasting diets
- Diet pills and liquids
- And others

We are bombarded with so many quick-fix solutions to our obesity epidemic, but do we really know the cost? We spend $50 billion a year on weight-loss products—but do we grasp their harmful effects on our bodies, minds, and moods?

* Notes
- Any restrictive or unbalanced diet can and will cause health issues and will only help you lose weight short-term. The key to good health & fitness is a balance between all the essential nutrients, including water, protein, carbohydrates, fats, vitamins and minerals. When you take one of these essentials out of the equation, you are asking for trouble.

- Diet pills, whether prescribed or over the counter, are basically stimulants that can be damaging to your health and cause dependency.
- When you go on a quick-fix program of eating special fake-food products, restricting certain nutrients, taking diet pills, or even starving yourself, you may lose some weight initially.
  - Rather than fat, however, you usually lose water weight and the weight you lose will return as soon as you go off that restrictive diet or stop taking the diet pills.
  - In many cases you will also gain back additional weight.
  - You will usually end up suffering physically, emotionally, and mentally, as well as driving your family and friends crazy.
- Any responsible diet program will never make you suffer or create health risks.
- Your weight can fluctuate daily—even up to five pounds—but genuine fat loss occurs over time. The average realistic and obtainable fat loss is anywhere from one-half to two pounds per week.
  - Losing fat the healthy and lasting way is a slow process, but you will love it when you reach your goals.
  - The best part of losing weight the right way is that there is a greater guarantee of fat loss and subsequent maintenance of your target body fat level, size, look, and mood.
- When you commit to a fitness program to lose body fat (whether through exercise, diet, or both) and you get results, you will need to stay on at least 65% to 75% of that program to maintain your desired physical condition.
- For lasting results, know that proper diet and exercise will have to be a part of your life forever! But when you make it part of a new lifestyle, it will be like taking a shower daily or brushing your teeth regularly—necessary, do-able, and even enjoyable.

* Restrictive and Unbalanced Diet Rules

- Never go on any type of quick-fix or extreme diet program and never take diet pills. In fact, run as fast as you can from them.
- Stick with a lifestyle plan like MY DIVA DIET and other programs based on sound nutrition and professional experience—you will never regret it.
- Fasting once in a while is acceptable, but it should be a juice fast for either cleansing or spiritual purposes.

- Make sure you are healthy enough for a fast.
- Fasting is not for fat loss, although you will lose water weight.
- Keep your fast to a few days to avoid losing muscle mass.

Factor #5: Exercise

32. Weekly exercise program

Americans' attitudes toward exercise reflect other values in our culture today: we have grown lazy and passive, expecting rewards to come to us without effort and hoping that others will do for us what we can and should do for ourselves. In terms of physical activity, the result is that our health & fitness levels have fallen dramatically.

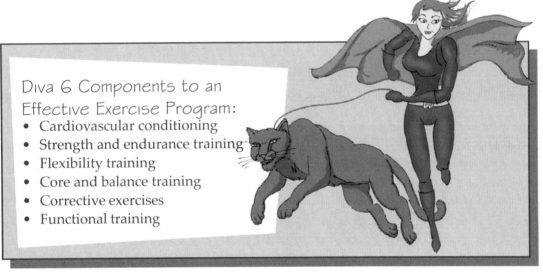

Diva 6 Components to an Effective Exercise Program:
- Cardiovascular conditioning
- Strength and endurance training
- Flexibility training
- Core and balance training
- Corrective exercises
- Functional training

* Notes
- The wide-ranging health benefits of regular exercise include:
  - Reducing the risk of heart disease, high blood pressure, osteoporosis, diabetes, and obesity
  - Helping keep joints, tendons, and ligaments flexible
  - Helping increase metabolism, energy, and endurance
  - Reducing some of the effects of aging
  - Contributing to mental well-being (including alleviating depression, stress, and anxiety) and ensuring better sleep

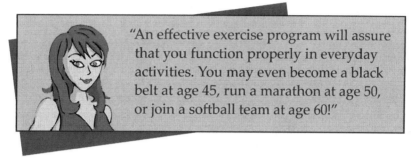

"An effective exercise program will assure that you function properly in everyday activities. You may even become a black belt at age 45, run a marathon at age 50, or join a softball team at age 60!"

- A properly designed and executed exercise program can improve or protect posture, help keep bones and muscles stronger, and maintain joints, tendons, and ligaments injury-free.
- Exercise can help improve your skin and enable your internal organs to function better.
- Exercise helps you lose body fat by:
  - Burning calories when you are exercising and increasing your metabolism for many hours afterward
  - Increasing your lean body mass, which:
    - Equals a higher sustained metabolic rate
    - Leads to a firmer, more sculptured physique
- Exercise makes you healthier, feel better, look younger and more alive—it's sexy!

* Exercise Rules
- There is only one main exercise rule when your goal is to lose fat and gain health: exercise is mandatory. So find something active you enjoy doing and make it part of your life right now.
- Exercise is crucial for fat loss and good health. It is also essential for maintaining low body fat and a fit physique. However, the frequency, duration, and intensity of your exercise will vary depending on your goals and other circumstances.
- Don't be extreme with your exercise program.

* A Quick Guide to Exercise
- The best thing to do when you've been cleared by your doctor and are ready to begin an exercise program is to hire a Certified Fitness Professional. That way you will not waste time, money, or risk injury.

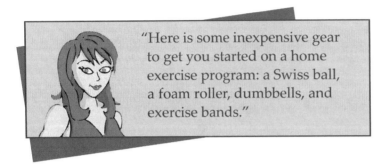

"Here is some inexpensive gear to get you started on a home exercise program: a Swiss ball, a foam roller, dumbbells, and exercise bands."

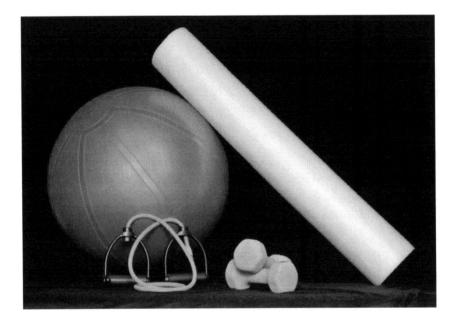

- An exercise program should consist of the six components shown in the following chart. Each workout should fit your age, current fitness level, and any medical or physical limitations you may have. Your goals, lifestyle, exercise interests, and commitment level should also be taken into consideration when your exercise program is designed.

Exercise Program Components

#1 Cardiovascular conditioning
- Purpose: Supports your heart and lungs, has many other health benefits; has a major impact on fat loss
- Types of activity:
  - Biking, running, fast walking, stair climbing, rowing, etc. (outside or on an indoor machine)
  - Consider: A spin class or a group aerobics class
- Frequency: 3 to 5 times per week
- Duration: Approximately 30 to 45 minutes
- Intensity: 75 to 85% of your maximum heart rate

#2 Strength and endurance training
- Purpose: Helps build muscle, strength and endurance, and bone density; has many other health benefits; increases lean body mass, which supports fat loss and makes you look firmer.
- Types of activity:
  - Weight training with free weights and some machines
  - Circuit training
  - Consider: Pilates, which covers some strength, core, and flexibility training
- Frequency: 3 to 5 times per week
- Duration: Approximately 30 to 45 minutes
- Intensity: Depends on the number of sets and repetitions, weight load, and the rest period between sets

#3 Flexibility training
- Purpose: Enhances your joints' ability to move through a full range of motion. Keeping your muscles flexible will help improve physical performance and posture and reduce the risk of injury, low back pain, and muscle soreness; increase the flow of blood and nutrients to tissues; and help improve muscle coordination. It not only will make you feel better but function better.
- Types of activity:
  - Stretching exercises (either alone or within a class setting)
  - Consider: A yoga class
- Frequency: 3 to 5 times per week (perhaps after an exercise program)
- Duration: Approximately 10 to 20 minutes (or more, if you have the time)
- Intensity: To the point of tightness, not pain

#4 Core and balance training
- Purpose: Supports the balanced development of the deep superficial muscles that stabilize, align, and move the trunk of the body, especially the abdominals and muscles of the back.
- Types of activity:
  - Core conditioning can be done with weights, exercise bands, medicine balls, or a Swiss ball (a large rubber ball used for exercise and physical therapy)
- Frequency, duration, and intensity: Core training can be incorporated into your exercise program (either with your weight training or in a class setting)

#5 Corrective exercises

- Purpose: Help improve posture and target ideal posture, defined as "that state of muscular and skeletal balance which protects the supporting structures of the body against injury or progressive deformity." It is during ideal posture that the muscles function most efficiently.
- Types of activity:
  - Exercises that help offset any muscle imbalances you may have developed through work injuries, sports, a poorly designed exercise program, or simple neglect. Corrective exercises help put your body back into its proper postural alignment so you not only function better but look and feel better. You can use weight training and flexibility techniques as well as a Swiss ball, foam rollers, and other modalities.
- Frequency, duration, and intensity: You can incorporate corrective exercises within your regular exercise routine, as long as they are tailored to your particular postural issues.

#6 Functional training

- Purpose: Improves functional movements that the body is engineered to do in everyday life—walking, running, climbing, lifting, bending, etc.— through a complex series of motions by several of the body's systems, including the nervous system, the muscular system, and the skeletal system.
  - These movements are important because they give us the ability to perform a variety of tasks—at work, at home, for recreation—now and in the future.
- Types of activity:
  - Functional training should be a part of your exercise program so that your body can do all the things it was meant to do—even at age 80!
- Frequency, duration, and intensity: You can fit your functional training into your weight training sessions.

Four Things for Women to Embrace with Exercise

#1 Sweating

- Sweating is good for you, so don't be concerned about how you look when you exercise—get moving and sweat when you work out!
- Sweating:
    - Speeds up metabolic processes of vital organs
    - Makes the heart pump hard, producing a drop in blood pressure
    - Strengthens the immune system and inhibits and kills bacteria and viruses
    - Relieves pain and speeds healing of joint injuries and other problems
    - Moves fluids through the body, thus cleansing the body and improving skin and cell function

#2 Muscle mass

- Muscle mass is great for your metabolic rate and makes you firmer.
- It is difficult for women to gain extreme amounts of muscle mass because we don't have the same hormonal make-up as men, so don't fear gaining too much muscle mass if you weight train.
    - If your exercise program is designed and executed properly and you are losing fat at the same rate of your muscle increase, you will not get bulky.

#3 Veins

- Veins are the blood vessels that carry blood to your heart. Visible veins (except for varicose veins) are a sign of good health, a signal of low body fat and lack of subcutaneous fluid. Don't consider them ugly but rather view them as a health & fitness measuring tool.

#4 Rest
- The health benefits of sleep include reducing inflammation, depression, and stress and increasing alertness, memory, immune function, and more.
  - Sleep also helps repair muscles after exercising, damage caused by stress, and harmful exposure to ultraviolet rays.
- Don't be extreme in your exercise program and be sure to get plenty of sleep and relaxation time.

✻ Exercise Resources
- Paul Chek of the Chek Institute
- ACE (American Council on Exercise)
- NESTA (National Exercise and Sports Trainers Association)

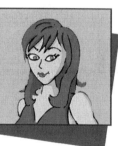

"For goodness' sake—take a break from your dieting and exercise regimen every 3 months or so. This is the last guideline in the MY DIVA DIET program!"

PART FIVE

The Menu Plan for Fat Loss

Every woman has the right to be beautiful.
~ Elizabeth Arden

Never eat more than you can lift.
~ Miss Piggy

Diva Daily Menu Plan
Phase One—Diva Reduction Outline

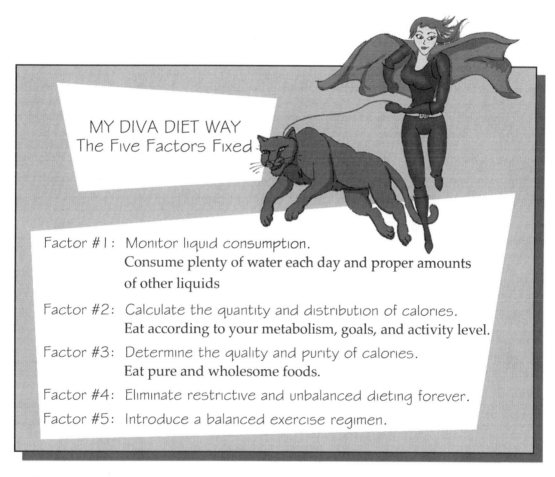

MY DIVA DIET WAY
The Five Factors Fixed

Factor #1: Monitor liquid consumption.
Consume plenty of water each day and proper amounts of other liquids

Factor #2: Calculate the quantity and distribution of calories.
Eat according to your metabolism, goals, and activity level.

Factor #3: Determine the quality and purity of calories.
Eat pure and wholesome foods.

Factor #4: Eliminate restrictive and unbalanced dieting forever.

Factor #5: Introduce a balanced exercise regimen.

Following the Diva Daily Menu Plan is a ten-week journey of fat loss and improved health. A ten-week investment (only two and one-half months) is not very long considering the trade off—to look, feel, and function better. This time frame will also help you make your dietary changes permanent.

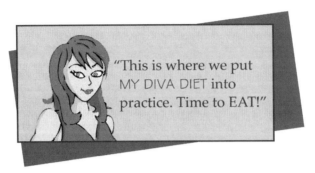

"This is where we put MY DIVA DIET into practice. Time to EAT!"

Your daily eating regimen:

- 1,200 to 1,300 calories per day
- 35% protein/45% carbs/20% fat
- Four to five meals per day every three to four hours
- Meal timing is up to your own individual schedule

Note on higher calorie intake for fat loss:

The 1,200 to 1,300 daily calorie range is for the average female to lose weight. Some of you may not need to go this low with your daily calories (see Paw Caloric Intake Guide—page 33). Your food choices will be the same; however, you can eat more. We recommend keeping your protein intake around 100 grams per day and fat intake at 30 grams; then eat more clean and pure carbohydrates. You should to eat your carbohydrate earlier in the day.

Your daily foods:

Paw Food Guide

- Clean and pure foods—natural, fresh, organic, and kosher
- Lean, healthy, fibrous, and *alive* foods
- Foods made by God (nature) for human consumption
- Carefully chosen man-made or man-manipulated foods

Diva Meal and Recipe Coding Design

The Diva Daily Menu Plan is broken down into four small meals per day to be eaten every three to four hours. Each of the daily four meals is labeled as a meal group.

- Each meal group is coded for your convenience.
- Each meal group has a targeted calorie and nutrient-breakdown guide for fat loss.
  - This way you end up with the proper calorie and nutrient totals at the end of each day.
  - This also is valuable when you want to create your own meal idea or substitution items within a meal.
- Each meal group has twelve meal ideas called Diva Reduction Meal (DRM) options with an option number (i.e., DRM #1).
  - The nutritional value for each DRM option is listed.

Some of the DRM options include Diva Reduction Recipes (not all Diva Reduction Recipes are in the DRM options). They are coded as well, and their nutritional value is listed individually within the DRM options and in the recipe section.

All meal options and recipes:

- Are for Phase One "Fat Reduction" and are healthy.
- Fit the MY DIVA DIET Food Criteria (Diva Reduction Pyramid—page 166).
- Are made with the Diva Reduction Good Food Choices At-a-Glance found in PART SIX.

Meals with Dairy Coding

Since MY DIVA DIET is low in dairy and we are sensitive to those of you who are lactose intolerant, we have labeled all DRM options and Diva Reduction Recipes that have dairy and/or dairy products (this does not include eggs).

- Dairy means from cattle, sheep, and goats.
- You can also substitute any dairy product with non-dairy items (like rice milk, soymilk, soy cheese, soy yogurt, soy butter, etc.).

Vegetarian Meal Coding

We have coded all DRM options and Diva Reduction Recipes that are pure vegetarian. This means they do not have any beef, fish, poultry, eggs, dairy, or dairy products.

Other Food Coding

DRM options and Diva Reduction Recipes that have eggs, fish, poultry, and beef are coded too.

If the following instructions are too complcated...just choose 4 meals from the Diva Reduction Meal Options (pgs. 167 to 181) each day. You will at least be in the Diva Reduction "ball park".

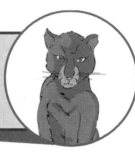

"Use the Diva Daily Menu Plan to improve health too!"

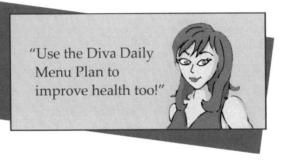

Diva Meal and Recipe Coding

Meal Group Codes and Targeted Calories with Nutrient Breakdowns for Fat Loss: Phase One—Diva Reduction) — Per meal group and daily

Breakfast
323 calories:
20 grams protein;
45 grams carbs; 7 grams fat

Lunch
343 calories:
35 grams protein;
35 grams carbs; 7 grams fat

Snack
254 calories:
15 grams protein;
35 grams carbs; 6 grams fat

Supper
370 calories:
40 grams protein;
25 grams carbs; 10 grams fat

Total Daily Nutrient Grams
- Based on 1,300 calories per day
- Protein: 113.8 grams
- Carbs: 146.3 grams
- Fat: 28.9 grams

Diva Reduction Meal Option Coding
- Within each of four meal groups are 12 Diva Reduction Meal (DRM) ideas that are labeled and numbered (i.e., DRM Option #1).
- Diva Reduction Recipes are labeled with an asterisk (*).

Special Food Codes Within the DRM Options and Diva Reduction Recipes

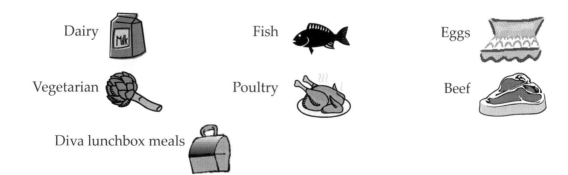

Dairy

Fish

Eggs

Vegetarian

Poultry

Beef

Diva lunchbox meals

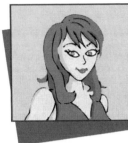

"You don't need to count calories! If you count your nutrient grams, you'll end up with the right daily calorie intake and your nutrient ratio will be accurate. My sidekick Paw helps keep me in line. You can use Paw's guide, below, to help keep you on track."

Paw Daily Nutrient Guide
Protein—Carbs—Fat

Diva Reduction Phase
Daily Nutrient Ratio =
35% protein/45% carbs/ 20% fat

Standard 1,300 Calories Per Day
- Protein = 113.8 grams
- Carbs = 146.3 grams
- Fat = 28.9 grams

Preferred Daily Range
- Protein = 100 to 120 grams
- Carbs = 130 to 150 grams
- Fat = 25 to 30 grams
- Fiber = 25 to 35 grams

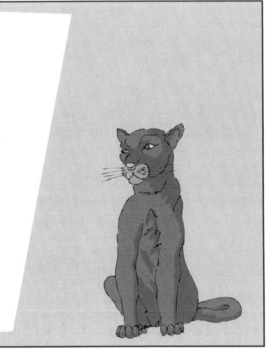

Food Values
MY DIVA DIET provides the nutritional value of each DRM option and Diva Reduction Recipe. Resources for nutritional values (food values) are compiled from the following:
- The actual food package of the item recommended
- Nutrition Advisor Mark Bricklyn in *Prevention Magazine*
- *The World's Healthiest Foods* by George Mateljan
- Calorie King website (www.calorieking.com)

Notes
- Nutritional value totals for each DRM option and Diva Reduction Recipe are approximate because many calorie counters vary in their calculations.
- Even though the DRM options' nutritional totals are approximate, they are very close to MY DIVA DIET recommendations. Some totals are a bit higher or lower due to the type of foods used for that particular DRM option.

The Numbers
- Each DRM option and Diva Reduction Recipe nutritional value total is listed in this order:
Total Calories/Protein grams/Carb grams/Fat grams/Fiber grams.
- Since we are BIG on the importance of fiber, the amount of fiber is listed in all of the DRM options and Diva Reduction Recipes. The milligrams of sodium are also listed in all of our recipes.

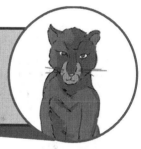

Think fiber—count your daily intake of fiber. For each meal you plan to eat, ask yourself this question, "Where's the fiber?" If the answer is none, it's probably not a good meal idea!

- We have done the math for you—you provide the discipline!
  - Some days you may be slightly over 1,300 calories and some days under 1,200 —that is okay. Just don't go under 1,000 or over 1,500 calories per day (unless you have determined you can lose weight with wholesome foods and higher calories).
  - If you want to be exact, add up your calories and nutrient totals at the end of each day. You can use the Food Diary Sheets in PART EIGHT.

- We have calculated the complete Diva Daily Menu Plan to end up close to 1,200 to 1,300 calories (totals are rounded to the nearest tenth to avoid confusion). If for some reason you have less than 1,200 calories at the end of the day, then you may eat a late-night snack to add another 50 to 200 calories.

- We also have made a variety of high- and low-calorie DRM options for those times when you are more hungry or less—you have the choice.

A margin of error has been factored into the total daily calories and daily nutrient ratios.

- 10% for calories = plus or minus 120 to 130 calories
- 15% for nutrient ratios = plus or minus
  - 15-18 grams of protein
  - 19-22 grams of carbohydrates
  - 3-5 grams of fat

This margin of error is designed for the following reasons:

- Possible deviations, alternatives and overages
- Portion mistakes
- Mixing and matching high and low calories
- Choosing too many vegetarian menu ideas
- Higher calorie liquid consumption
- Cheat days

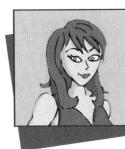

"Try to stick to the calories and nutrient ratio recommended. But we know how life is, so we have provided some leeway—that way you are more apt to stay on the program for more than a few weeks!"

Diva Daily Menu Plan
Phase One—Diva Reduction Instructions

Liquid Intake

- Water should be consumed all day every day.

- In order to avoid adding too many extra calories to your day, keep your liquid consumption to tea and coffee (plain, which has no calories).

- Milk (whether dairy, soy or rice) does contain calories, so keep these items to a minimum.

- Fresh juice (fruit or vegetable) and meal replacement drinks have quite a few calories. Monitor these so your daily totals won't go too high.

- Lastly, if you decide to keep drinking liquids that are not conducive to getting lean and healthy—like high-fat, high-sugar coffees and teas, soda (diet or not), sugary drinks, non-fresh juice, poor-quality meal replacement drinks, and alcohol—you can expect poor results.

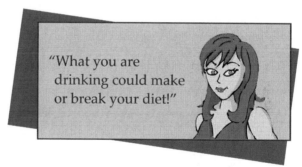

"What you are drinking could make or break your diet!"

Choosing Diva Reduction Meal (DRM) Options

- It is best to choose one DRM option from each of the four meal groups every day to equal four balanced meals per day (and a fifth snack if needed).

- You can have different DRM options within the four meal groups each day for variety.

- It is also a good idea to keep the meal groups in order (i.e., breakfast, lunch, snack, supper). OR, if you have an early breakfast, you may need to follow with a snack, then lunch, and an early supper.

- Put your snacks (one or two) where you need to—those times when it has been three hours since your last meal or it will be three hours until your next meal.

161

- On occasion during a given day, you may choose two DRM options from a particular meal group you like—just make sure you end up with four balanced meals per day. For example, if you like eggs, you may have an egg option in the morning then again for lunch.
- You can change around the breakfast, lunch, and snack meal groups but not the supper meal group.
  - The Supper Restriction
    - Supper is reserved for lean protein and veggies, and maybe some fruit.
    - Legumes, nuts, and seeds are fine for for supper too.
    - Occasionally you can have grains or grain products for supper.
    - You can put the supper meal group anywhere in your day, just try not to eat breakfast, lunch, and snack meal groups at night unless you make the appropriate adjustments to ensure the meal is light, lean, and full of fresh veggies.

Meal Timing

The time of the day at which you choose to eat is an individual decision—it depends first on your wake-up and bedtime schedule. Other factors that determine when you eat your meals include family, work, social activities, exercise timing, etc. Here are some simple guidelines to help:
- Time your meals every three to four hours after you have eaten your first meal.
- Try to eat supper about three hours before bedtime.
- A light late-night snack an hour or so before bedtime is okay.

Exceptions to Choosing

- Choose only one to two DRM options that have dairy in them (each day)—that way you stick with a diet low in dairy.
  - Keeping in line with low dairy also keeps your cheese consumption in check, which means your fat grams have a better chance of staying within the low-fat guidelines of 30 grams per day or less.

> If you want to lose fat a little quicker limit your use of dairy and dairy products to once or twice per month.

- Choose only two all-vegetarian DRM options each day. That way you get enough protein and you won't go over on carbohydrates.
  - The exception is when you are having an "all-vegetarian" day.
- Choose only one beef DRM option per month.

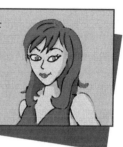

"Grass-fed beef is a good source of protein, vitamins B12 and B6, iron, zinc, niacin, and phosphorus; however, there are problems with beef that should be addressed."

Here are some things to consider about beef:

1. Over consumption
2. The quality of the beef
3. The cut of beef
4. High fat (saturated) and cholesterol content
5. How the cattle are raised and slaughtered
6. The condition and practices of the companies that process and package beef (this also applies to other animal meats, like poultry and lamb).

Desserts

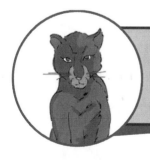

Try a tangerine or an orange for dessert (as Japanese restaurants do). It will make you full without making you fat.

Substitutions

- You can also substitute your own food items within the DRM options if they fit the MY DIVA DIET Food Criteria (Diva Reduction Pyramid) and are close to the targeted calorie and nutrient breakdown for each meal group provided at the beginning of this section.

- Since fruits and veggies are seasonal and we all have different tastes, feel free to change them according to your preference within the DRM option. The calories won't change that much (except for high calories in an avocado). Just make sure the portion is the same.

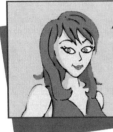

"In choosing foods for your substitutions and meal ideas, use the Golden Food Rule: If God (nature) made it, it is safe. If it is man-made, it must be examined thoroughly!"

Making Your Own Reduction Meals and Recipes:

- Use the Diva Reduction Pyramid (PART TWO and PART FIVE)
- Use the Diva Reduction Good Food Choices At-a-Glance (PART SIX)
- Try to stay close to the targeted calorie and nutrient breakdown for each meal group—breakfast, lunch, snacks, and supper.
- Use the following guides to ensure that your meal ideas and recipes are made for fat reduction.

Paw Guide for Diva Reduction Meals and Recipes
(Per Meal & Recipe)

- Calories = 100 to 400
- Protein = No more than 40 grams
- Carbs = No more than 55 grams
- Fat = No more than 10 grams
- Fiber = More is better here
  (5 to 10 grams per meal)
- Sodium = No more than double the amount of calories (less is better)
  (i.e. 100 calories = 100-200 miligrams sodium)

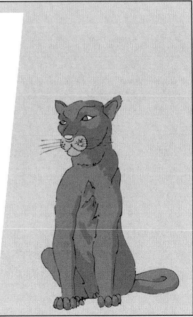

Note for Extra-Lean Divas: Stay strict with the MY DIVA DIET Program and use this Paw Guide and Paw Tip.

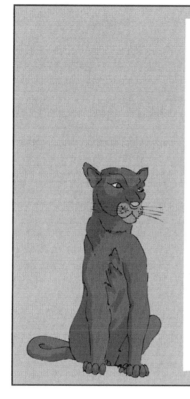

Paw Extra-Lean Diva Guide

- Egg whites only
- Non-fat dairy and dairy products
- No cheese and butter
- No mayonnaise, sauces, dips and watch the condiments
- Plain balsamic vinegar for salad dressing
- Olive oil, avocados, nuts, and seeds are great, but in small amounts

----

* With these simple adjustments and eating lean fish and poultry daily, while keeping your beef intake to once per month or less, you will average about 20 grams of fat per day.

Fat is not the only thing you can reduce to be an Extra-Lean Diva. Eliminate or decrease your intake of ALL:
- Sugar and extra sweeteners
- Dairy and dairy products
- Cheat Days

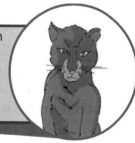

Phase One: Diva Reduction Pyramid
(MY DIVA DIET Food Criteria)

1,200 to 1,300 Calories
Per Day (Average)—For 10 weeks

- 35% protein/45% carbs/20% fat
- 4 to 5 meals per day
- Clean and pure foods
- Natural, fresh, organic, and kosher foods

- High in water intake
- High in nutrients
- High in antioxidants
- High in real/live pure organic foods
- High in alkaline-forming foods (low acidic-forming)
- High in the proper balance of protein, carbs, and fat
- High in fiber

- Alcohol-free
- Flourless/white flour-free
- Wheat-free, partially gluten-free
- Free of artificial ingredients
- Free of genetically modified foods
- Junk food-free

- Extremely low to no processed and refined foods
- Extremely low in food additives and preservatives
- Naturally low-glycemic

- Extra low dairy
- Extra low sugar
- Extra low sodium
- Extra low in saturated fats and cholesterol

Diva Reduction Meal Options
* Indicates a Diva Recipe. See next section for recipes.

Option #1
Diva Spicy Scramble*
with Tortillas and Fruit

*122 calories
16.6 g protein
3.1 g carbs
5.2 g fat
1 g fiber
+ 2 corn sprouted tortillas, warmed
+ 1 cup strawberries

- - - - - - - - - - - -

287 calories
20.5 g protein
36.6 g carbs
7.8 g fat
7.9 g fiber

Option #2
Diva Power Omelet*
with Potato and Fruit

*174 calories
25 g protein
5.7 g carbs
5.4 g fat
1 g fiber
+4 oz. Yukon gold potato, baked or boiled
+ 1/2 cup melon

- - - - - - - - - - - -

340 calories
28.8 g protein
44.6 g carbs
6 g fat
3.4 g fiber
Notes: Replace cottage cheese with soy cheese to make a non-dairy meal.

Option #3
Diva Frittata*
with Rice and Berries

*172 calories
20 g protein
6 g carbs
7.2 g fat
2.2 g fiber
+ 1/4 cup white, brown or wild rice,
cooked, plain
+ 1 cup blackberries (raspberries and
blueberries are great, too)
- - - - - - - - - - - -
301.5 calories
22.3 g protein
35.9 g carbs
8.2 g fat
9.4 g fiber

Option #4
Diva Pineapple Pleasure*
with Side of Fruit

*181 calories
15.4 g protein
27.8 g carbs
1 g fat
1.8 g fiber
+ 1 medium apple
- - - - - - - - - - - -
262 calories
15.7 g protein
48.9 g carbs
1.5 g fat
4.8 g fiber

Option #5
Egg White Omelet with
Veggies and Side of Fruit

3 egg whites, plain
1/2 cup veggies (like mushrooms,
onions, and 1/4 avocado)
Cook veggies with egg whites
+ 4 oz. potato, baked or boiled
+ 1 cup diced cantaloupe
- - - - - - - - - - - -
300.5 calories
16.7 g protein
46.3 g carbs
6.5 g fat
6.1 g fiber

Option #6
Hard-boiled Eggs
with Potato and Fruit

1 hard-boiled egg
plus 1 hard-boiled egg white
+ 4 oz. potato (baked or boiled), topped
with salsa
+ 1 whole grapefruit (or orange)
- - - - - - - - - - - -
279 calories
13.7 g protein
45.3 g carbs
5.7 g fat
2.5 g fiber

Option #7
Hot Cereal and Fruit

3/4 to 1 cup cooked
oatmeal (1/2 cup dry = 1 cup cooked)
+ 1/2 cup low-fat milk
+ 1/2 piece fruit of your choice
Notes: If you want, skip the fruit and
add 1 tsp. honey or agave nectar in your
oatmeal

- - - - - - - - - - - -

with fruit
272 calories
10.9 g protein
48.2 g carbs
5 g fat
5.9 g fiber

 Notes: Replace milk with soy or
rice milk to make a vegetarian
meal

Option #8
Hot Cereal, Yogurt, and
Fruit

3/4 to 1 cup cooked oatmeal,
quinoa, or other grain like buckwheat or
amaranth
(1/2 cup dry = 1 cup cooked)
+ 1/2 cup plain low-fat yogurt
+ 1/2 cup fresh berries (blackberries,
blueberries, raspberries, strawberries)

- - - - - - - - - - - -

324 calories
14.5 g protein
54 g carbs
6.4 g fat
8.5 g fiber

 Notes: Replace with soy yogurt
to make a non-dairy and
vegetarian meal

 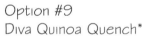

Option #9
Diva Quinoa Quench*

- - - - - - - - - - - -

***374 calories**
14 g protein
52 g carbs
12.5 g fat
6.5 g fiber
Notes: This has plenty of calories.
Eliminate the almonds for lower fat.

Option #10
Hot Cereal and Fruit

1 cup cooked cream of rice cereal
+ 1/2 cup rice milk
+ 1/2 mango (1 cup) or fruit of your
choice

- - - - - - - - - - - -

254 calories
2.9 g protein
57.8 g carbs
1.5 g fat
2.3 g fiber

Option #11
Cold Cereal and Fruit

Option #12
Diva Meal Replacement
Drinks*

1 cup cold cereal
(like Erewhon Crispy Brown Rice)
+ 1/2 cup low-fat milk
+ 1 whole banana

- - - - - - - - - - - -

276 calories
7.2 g protein
56.7 g carbs
3.5 g fat
3 g fiber

Notes: Replace milk with soy or rice milk to make a vegetarian meal

Diva Smoothie*

- - - - - - - - - - - -

***175 calories**
5.4 g protein
35.5 g carbs
2.6 g fat
13.4 g fiber

Diva Protein Shake*

- - - - - - - - - - - -

***334.5 calories**
24 g protein
58 g carbs
1.6 g fat
10 g fiber

Diva Veggie Drink*

- - - - - - - - - - - -

***200 calories**
8.8 g protein
39.6 g carbs
0.8 g fat
12 g fiber
Notes: These liquid meals can be used for any meal.

Option #1
Chicken Breast
with Salad and Rice

4 oz. plain chicken breast, grilled
On or with small mixed green salad
+ 1 Tbsp. low-fat, low-sugar dressing or vinegar/olive oil
+ 1/2 cup brown or white rice, steamed, plain
- - - - - - - - - - - -
352.8 calories
39.5 g protein
32.7 g carbs
6 g fat
2.5 g fiber

Option #2
Chicken Ceasar Salad

3 oz. plain chicken breast, grilled
On 3 cups romaine lettuce
+ 1 Tbsp. Parmesan cheese
+ 1 Tbsp. low-fat Caesar dressing
- - - - - - - - - - - -
309.3 calories
41.3 g protein
6.1 g carbs
11.9 g fat
3 g fiber

Option #3
Diva Spinach Salad*
with Chicken and Melon

*140.5 calories**
9.3 g protein
8.6 g carbs
7.3 g fat
2.5 g fiber
+ 2 oz. plain chicken breast, grilled
+ 2 cups watermelon cubes
- - - - - - - - - - - -
337.1 calories
28.1 g protein
31.6 g carbs
10.8 g fat
3.7 g fiber

Option #4
Grilled Turkey Patty
with Sliced Tomatoes and
Cucumbers

4 oz. plain, lean ground turkey, grilled
+ 2 sliced tomatoes
+ 1 sliced cucumber
+ balsamic vinegar as dressing
+ 1/2 mango
- - - - - - - - - - - -
363 calories
28.8 g protein
44.6 g carbs
9.5 g fat
10 g fiber

Option #5
Diva Tuna Mixture*
with Corn Cakes
and Chickpeas

1/2 to 3/4 cup
*216.7 calories
32.5 g protein
3.7 g carbs
7.7 g fat
0.5 g fiber
On 3 corn cakes or 1 rice cake and
topped with 1/4 cup chickpeas
- - - - - - - - - - - -

358.2 calories
36.5 g protein
33.3 g carbs
8.4 g fat
4.5 g fiber
Notes:
•For lower calories, skip the rice cakes
and chickpeas and eat tuna mixture over
butterhead lettuce along with 1/2 cup
applesauce.
•You can also make your own tuna
mixture or salad.

 Option #6
Fresh Fish
with Salad and Rice

4 oz. plain trout, grilled (or other fresh
fish)
On or with large mixed green salad or
any raw vegetable salad
+ 1 tsp. low-fat, low-sugar dressing or
other low-fat Italian dressing
+ 1/2 cup wild rice, steamed, plain
- - - - - - - - - - - - -

348.6 calories
36.6 g protein
29.9 g carbs
9.1 g fat
5.5 g fiber

 Option #7
Diva Baked Potato*

- - - - - - - - - - - - -
*335.5 calories
9 g protein
54.2 g carbs
9 g fat
4.2 g fiber
Notes: This is great for when you need
an extra carbohydrate boost.

 Option #8
Diva Beet and Chicken
Salad*

- - - - - - - - - - - - -
*360 calories
33.2 g protein
31.5 g carbs
9.5 g fat
8.3 g fiber

Option #9
Beans and Rice

A) 1/2 cup of any legume (kidney beans, chickpeas, lima, navy, or pinto) + 1/2 cup brown or wild rice, steamed, plain

- - - - - - - - - - - - -

221.4 calories
10.2 g protein
43.2 g carbs
1.4 g fat
7.7 g fiber

B) **Diva 3-Bean Dish***
 3/4 cup

- - - - - - - - - - - - -

***206 calories**
8.9 g protein
33.1 g carbs
5.2 g fat
9.3 g fiber
Notes: Top both option A & B with some fresh salsa or use Diva Salsa*

Option #10
Diva Onion Soup*
with Turkey and Salad

1 small serving
***86.5 calories**
4 g protein
8.1 g carbs
4.1 g fat
1.5 g fiber
+ 3 oz. plain chicken or turkey breast, grilled
+ salad of 1/2 medium cucumber, 1 diced tomato, and 1 cup shredded carrot
+ 1 to 2 Tbsp. balsamic vinegar as dressing

- - - - - - - - - - - - -

324.3 calories
33.7 g protein
29.2 g carbs
8.1 g fat
9 g fiber
Notes: Soup is the best fast food—quick to eat, easy to digest, and full of veggies.

Option #11
Amy's Organic Lentil
Soup (gluten-free) with
Spelt Cakes and Plums

1 cup
150 calories
8 g protein
19 g carbs
4.5 g fat
9 g fiber
+ 2 spelt cakes
+ 2 small plums

- - - - - - - - - - - - -

273 calories
11 g protein
46.2 g carbs
5.5 g fat
13 g fiber
Notes: You can replace this with any
gluten-free, low-sodium, low-sugar,
organic vegetable soup.

Option #12
Diva Vegetarian Tostada*
with Side of Fruit

*228 calories**
10 g protein
38.2 g carbs
7.6 g fat
12.9 g fiber
+ 1/2 of a papaya

- - - - - - - - - - - - -

287 calories
10.9 g protein
53.1 g carbs
7.8 g fat
15.5 g fiber

Option #1
Yam or Sweet Potato

1 large yam or sweet potato with skin, baked or boiled
+ 1 tsp. cinnamon
- - - - - - - - - - - - -
234 calories
4 g protein
55.4 g carbs
0.2 g fat
6.8 g fiber
Notes: If using 1 Tbsp. butter instead of cinnamon, add 70 calories and 7 g fat

Option #2
Hummus and Rice Cakes
with Veggies

3 Tbsp. hummus
+ 2 rice cakes (spread hummus on them like a dip)
+ 1 tomato dressed with balsamic vinegar
- - - - - - - - - - - - -
256 calories
6.1 g protein
44.5 g carbs
5.7 g fat
5.1 g fiber

Option #3
Tortilla Wrap

2 sprouted corn tortillas, warmed
+ 1 Tbsp. reduced-fat cream cheese
+ 1 1/2 cup veggies (lettuce, tomato, cucumber, radish)
+ 1 cup honeydew melon cubes
Notes: Spread cream cheese on tortilla and then add veggies, like a burrito or wrap.
- - - - - - - - - - - - -
232 calories
7.5 g protein
41.9 g carbs
5.4 g fat
8.3 g fiber

Option #4
Mochi, Cottage Cheese,
and Fruit

1 (2-inch) cooked mochi square
+ 1/2 cup low-fat cottage cheese
+ 1 cup watermelon cubes
Notes: Scoop cottage cheese in the middle of cooked mochi square to make a creamy and gooey nutritious snack.
- - - - - - - - - - - - -
253 calories
17 g protein
39.6 g carbs
2.9 g fat
3.6 g fiber

Option #5
Avocado, Carrot, and
Tomato Salad

1/2 medium avocado, 1 sliced tomato
and 1 shredded carrot
+ balsamic or rice vinegar as dressing
+ 3 fresh apricots
- - - - - - - - - - - - -

270 calories
3.8 g protein
31.6 g carbs
16.3 g fat
8 g fiber
Notes: This option is high in fat (half of
your daily allowance when reducing
body fat), so make sure the rest of your
fat intake for the day is low.

Option #7
Dried Fruit and Cheese

4 organic dried figs (or other
dried fruit like prunes or dates)
+ 2 pieces reduced-fat string cheese
- - - - - - - - - - - - -

246 calories
13.3 g protein
36.7 g carbs
5 g fat
6.7 g fiber
Notes: Use 2 oz. soy cheese to make it a
vegetarian meal

Option #6
Nuts, Soy Yogurt, and
Berries

1 oz. (2 Tbsp.) almonds or other nuts
+ 3/4 cup (6 oz.) plain soy yogurt
+ 1/2 cup blueberries
- - - - - - - - - - - - -

285.5 calories
8 g protein
41.8 g carbs
9.8 g fat
4.2 g fiber
Notes: This option is high in fat, so
make sure the rest of your fat intake for
the day is low.

Option #8
Rice Cakes with Cream
Cheese or Nut Butter

2 rice cakes or 6 thin corn cakes
Spread with 2 Tbsp. reduced-fat
cream cheese
Or 1 Tbsp. almond or nut butter
- - - - - - - - - - - - -

Cream Cheese
210 calories
4 g protein
34 g carbs
7 g fat
2 g fiber

Nut Butter
245 calories
6 g protein
35 g carbs
8 g fat
3 g fiber

Option #9
Popcorn, Cheese, and
Fruit

A) 2 cups plain air-popped popcorn
+ 1 piece string cheese or 1 oz.
mozzarella
+ 1 cup grapes
- - - - - - - - - - - - -
200 calories
9.3 g protein
29.2 g carbs
6.9 g fat
3 g fiber

B) 2 cups plain air-popped popcorn
+ 2 slices American soy cheese
+ 1 medium apple
- - - - - - - - - - - - -
223 calories
8.3 g protein
34.5 g carbs
6 g fat
5.4 g fiber

Option #11
Fruit and Cottage
Cheese

1 large papaya
+ 1/2 cup low-fat cottage cheese
Notes: Eat separately or scoop cottage
cheese into papaya.
- - - - - - - - - - - - -
200 calories
15.8 g protein
32.9 g carbs
1.6 g fat
5.2 g fiber

Option #10
Fruit and Nut Butter

1 apple or banana
+ 1 Tbsp. natural peanut butter
+ 2 prunes or dates
Notes: Spread nut butter on apple or
banana.
- - - - - - - - - - - - -
250 calories
5.6 g protein
39.5 g carbs
8.5 g fat
5.2 g fiber

Option #12
Celery, Nut Butter, and
Fruit

5 to 6 celery sticks
+ 1 Tbsp. nut butter
+ 1 large peach
+ 1 (1/2 oz.) miniature box of raisins
Notes: Spread nut butter on celery and
enjoy a healthy, creamy snack with
crunch.
- - - - - - - - - - - - -
224 calories
7 g protein
32.6 g carbs
8.6 g fat
6.9 g fiber

Option #1
Salmon with Veggies

4 oz. salmon, grilled or poached
+ 1 1/2 cup steamed broccoli
+ 1 artichoke
- - - - - - - - - - - - -
381.3 calories
41.6 g protein
25.5 g carbs
13.5 g fat
7.5 g fiber
Note: This option is high in essential fats.

Option #2
Trout or Snapper with
Corn on the Cobb and
Cucumbers

5 oz. trout or snapper, grilled or poached
+ 1 corn on cob, steamed, plain
+ 1 sliced cucumber dressed with balsamic vinegar
- - - - - - - - - - - - -
328.3 calories
42 g protein
28.1 g carbs
4.5 g fat
5.9 g fiber

Option #3
Fresh Fish with
Salad and Veggies

4 oz. trout or other fresh fish, grilled or poached
+ 1 to 2 cups mixed green salad
+ 1 to 2 Tbsp. low-fat Italian dressing
+ 1 1/2 cups zucchini, steamed
- - - - - - - - - - - - -
307.6 calories
34.9 g protein
22.9 g carbs
8.9 g fat
7.9 g fiber

Option #4
Diva Chicken Veggie
Stir-Fry* with Edamame

*246.5 calories
34.5 g protein
23.6 g carbs
3.1 g fat
6.3 g fiber
+ 20 Edamame
- - - - - - - - - - - - -
306.5 calories
39.7 g protein
28 g carbs
5.9 g fat
7.9 g fiber

Option #5
Chicken Breast with
Veggies and Spinach
Salad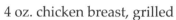

4 oz. chicken breast, grilled
+ 2 steamed carrots
+ 1 cup spinach salad with 1 Tbsp. olive
oil and vinegar or light Italian dressing,
topped with 1 Tbsp. feta cheese
- - - - - - - - - - - - -
369 calories
44.4 g protein
24 g carbs
10.7 g fat
8.6 g fiber
Note: Eliminate feta cheese to reduce
calories, fat and make a non-dairy meal.

Option #6
Turkey Breast with
Sauteed Veggies and
Salad

4 oz. turkey breast,
grilled or baked
+ 1 cup grilled or sautéed bell peppers,
onions, and mushrooms
+ 1 cup grilled eggplant
+ small green salad with low fat
dressing
- - - - - - - - - - - - -
324.3 calories
41 g protein
29.8 g carbs
4.9 g fat
8.8 g fiber

Option #7
Diva Bean Taco Salad*

- - - - - - - - - - - - -
*273 calories
12.5 g protein
38 g carbs
9.6 g fat
10 g fiber

Option #8
Diva Spicy Chicken Soup*
with Veggies

*284 calories
31.5 g protein
28.8 g carbs
4.3 g fat
3.9 g fiber
+ 1 cup cooked cauliflower
- - - - - - - - - - - - -
312 calories
33.7 g protein
33.8 g carbs
4.9 g fat
7.3 g fiber

Option #9
Diva Turkey Patty* with
Diva Garlic Pepper Sauté*

Option #10
Diva Special No-Bun
Burger* with Veggies

*185 calories
22 g protein
7 g carbs
7 g fat
0 g fiber

- - - - - - - - - - - -

*164 calories
9.2 g protein
28.2 g carbs
3.1 g fat
6.1 g fiber

- - - - - - - - - - - -

*349 calories
31.2 g protein
35.2 g carbs
10.1 g fat
6.1 g fiber

Notes: To make a vegetarian
meal, make a side salad and skip
the turkey patty

*305 calories
38.5 g protein
9.9 g carbs
15.3 g fat
2.3 g fiber
+1 cup Brussels sprouts
Or 1/2 cup butternut squash

- - - - - - - - - - - -

Brussels sprouts
365 calories
42.5 g protein
23.5 g carbs
16.1 g fat
9.1 g fiber

Butternut squash
346 calories
39.4 g protein
20.6 g carbs
15.4 g fat
5.2 g fiber
Notes: This option is a high-fat choice.
To make a non-dairy meal, skip the
feta cheese in the Diva Special No-Bun
Burger recipe. Lean ground beef is also
an option to make these no-bun burgers.

Option #11
Beef of Choice with
Asparagus and Beets

4 oz. lean beef, grilled (filet,
flank, New York, rib-eye, sirloin)
+ 8 spears asparagus, steamed
+ 1 beet, boiled
- - - - - - - - - - - - -

301.6 calories
36.2 g protein
13.5 g carbs
11.5 g fat
1.5 g fat
1.7 g fiber
Notes: Beef option should be kept to
once a month.

Option #12
Beef of Choice with
Veggies

4 oz. lean beef, grilled (filet,
flank, New York, rib-eye, sirloin)
+ 1/2 cup green beans, steamed
+ 1/2 cup cauliflower, steamed
- - - - - - - - - - - - -

255 calories
26.9 g protein
12.5 g carbs
10.8 g fat
7.7 g fiber
Notes: Beef option should be kept to
once a month.

Diva Reduction Recipes
"Fit Meals in Minutes"
"Combining quick and convenient with sound nutrition!"

MY DIVA DIET knows how busy women are these days. We try to balance families and friends, church, pets, household, cleaning, and grocery shopping. Then we have our careers, creative ideas, our looks, etc. The younger generation of women and teenagers try to do it all, too—juggling parents, stepparents, grandparents, siblings, pets, school, friends, sports, hobbies, and parties. As women we are often so busy that we put our health & fitness last, including our abilities to cook and eat healthy meals. This, however, is something we need to change—we need to re-prioritize.

Because we truly want you to succeed with MY DIVA DIET, we have designed quick Diva Recipes that meet the criteria for fat reduction as well as sound nutritional guidelines. You don't have to give up taste when you eat correctly. In fact, you will learn that wholesome and fit foods taste better than junk food.

NOTE: The Diva Meal and Recipe Coding is used in the Diva Reduction Recipes. Not all recipes are used in the Diva Reduction Meal options.

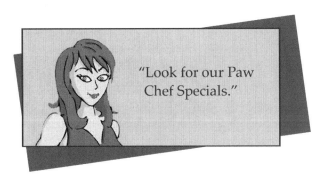

"Look for our Paw Chef Specials."

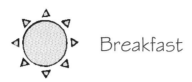 Breakfast

Diva Spicy Scramble

1 whole egg + 2 egg whites
1/2 cup mushrooms, sliced
2 Tbsp. yellow onion, chopped
1/2 Serrano chili pepper, diced
black pepper to garnish
non-stick cooking spray

Preparation: Whip together egg and egg whites in a small bowl, set aside. Spray a skillet with non-stick spray and heat over medium-low heat. Add mushrooms and sauté 2 to 4 minutes until soft. Add onion and chili pepper and cook for another minute. Add eggs and black pepper and stir into a scramble, another 2 to 4 minutes or until eggs are desired consistency.

Makes 1 Serving
Nutritional Value: 122 calories; 16.6 g protein; 3.1 g carbs; 5.2 g fat; 1 g fiber; 182 mg sodium

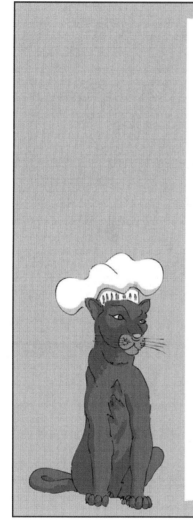

Diva Frittata

2 whole eggs + 5 egg whites
1/4 cup onion, chopped
1/2 cup mushrooms, diced
1/2 cup raw spinach
non-stick cooking spray
1 Tbsp. Parmesan cheese, grated

Preparation: Pre-heat the oven to 450 degrees. Whip together eggs and egg whites in a bowl. Spray a skillet with non-stick spray and cook veggies on medium heat until *al dente*. Spray a square baking pan with non-stick spray and pour in eggs and cooked veggies. Top with freshly grated Parmesan cheese. Place in pre-heated oven. Cook until firm, about 15 minutes or until desired texture.

Makes 2 Servings —
Recommended Serving Size: 1/2 of the frittata
Nutritional Value per serving: 172 calories;
20 g protein; 6 g carbs; 7.2 g fat; 2.2 g fiber;
346 mg sodium

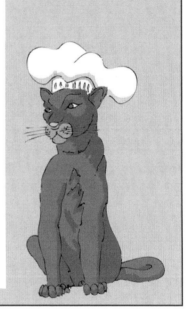

Diva Power Omelet

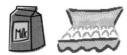

1 whole egg + 2 egg whites
1 Tbsp. onion, chopped
2 medium mushrooms, sliced
1/4 tomato, diced
1/4 cup cottage cheese
non-stick cooking spray

Preparation: Whip egg, egg whites, and vegetables in a bowl. Spray a skillet with non-stick spray and heat on medium heat. Pour in egg and veggie mixture and cook 2 to 3 minutes, and then flip over with a spatula. Scoop cottage cheese onto omelet, and then fold in half. Turn off stove and place lid on top of skillet to allow cottage cheese to melt somewhat.

Makes 1 Serving
Nutritional Value: 174 calories; 25 g protein; 5.7 g carbs; 5.4 g fat;
1 g fiber; 450 mg sodium

Diva Golden Omelet

1 whole egg + 2 egg whites
1/2 Roma tomato, chopped
4 asparagus tips, cooked and chopped into small pieces
1 Tbsp. Romano cheese, grated
non-stick cooking spray

Preparation: Whip together egg and egg whites in a bowl. Spray skillet with non-stick spray and heat on medium heat or use "eggie pan." Pour eggs in heated skillet or "eggie pan" and arrange tomatoes, asparagus, and cheese on top. When bottom of egg is cooked, fold in half with the fillings inside. Continue cooking until desired consistency is reached.

Makes 1 Serving
Nutritional Value: 151 calories; 16.8 g protein; 4.7 g carbs; 6.6 g fat;
1.1 g fiber; 258.5 mg sodium

Diva Cabbage and Carrot Omelet

1 whole egg + 2 egg whites
1/4 cup packaged cabbage, carrot blend
non-stick cooking spray

Preparation: Whip together egg, egg whites, and cabbage carrot blend in a bowl. Spray skillet or "eggie pan" with non-stick spray and heat on medium heat. Pour in egg and veggie blend and cook for about 10 minutes or until desired consistency is reached.

Makes 1 Serving
Nutritional Value: 109 calories; 13.7 g protein; 0.8 g carbs; 5.1 g fat;
0.3 g fiber; 183.3 mg sodium

Diva Quinoa Quench

1 cup cooked quinoa
1 oz. almonds, chopped
1 oz. raisins
1/2 cup low-fat organic milk

Preparation: Cook quinoa as directed on package in a saucepan or rice cooker. Combine cooked quinoa, almonds, and raisins in a bowl and top with milk.

Makes 1 Serving
Nutritional Value: 374 calories; 14 g protein; 52 g carbs; 12.5 g fat;
6.5 g fiber; 60 mg sodium

 Notes: To make this recipe vegetarian, use soy or rice milk.

Diva Pineapple Pleasure

2 pineapple rings, in juice or fresh
1/2 cup low-fat organic cottage cheese
2 corn thins (your choice of flaxseed, soy or other flavor)

Preparation: In a skillet, grill pineapple rings on medium heat for 2 minutes. Place each grilled pineapple ring on top of each corn thin. Top with cottage cheese.

Makes 1 Serving
Nutritional Value: 181 calories; 15.4 g protein; 27.8 g carbs; 1 g fat;
1.8 g fiber; 329 mg sodium

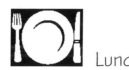 Lunch

High-Fiber, High-Potassium Diva Three-Bean Dish

1/2 cup chickpeas
1/2 cup kidney beans
1/2 cup black beans
1/2 cup red onion, diced
3 tomatoes, diced
3 Tbsp. Balsamic vinaigrette dressing

Preparation: Mix together all ingredients and enjoy!

Makes 3 to 4 Servings — Recommended Serving Size: 3/4 cup
Nutritional Value Per Serving: 206 calories; 8.9 g protein; 33.1 g carbs; 5.2 g fat;
9.3 g fiber; 292 mg sodium; 616.3 mg potassium
Notes: Use low sodium canned beans and rinse them in water to remove excess
sodium.

Diva Baked Potato in Less Than an Hour

1 medium-large baking potato
1/2 cup broccoli, chopped
1 Tbsp. Parmesan, grated
1 Tbsp. whipped butter
1/2 Tbsp. parsley, chopped

Preparation: Bake pierced potato in 400-degree oven for 40 to 50 minutes. Just before
potato is done, in small saucepan boil 1/2 quart water and boil broccoli for 1 to 3
minutes, until tender. Strain broccoli and add it to opened potato; then add all other
toppings and serve.

Makes 1 Serving
Nutritional Value: 335.5 calories; 9 g protein; 54.2 g carbs; 9 g fat;
4.2 g fiber; 211 mg sodium
Notes: For a quicker recipe, use last night's boiled potato. Re-heat it for about 10
minutes and follow the same instructions.

Diva Veggie Rice Stir-Fry

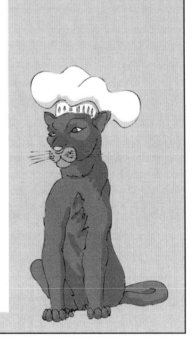

1/2 cup brown rice
1/2 cup broccoli, chopped
1/2 cup mushrooms, sliced
1/2 cup yellow onions, chopped
1/2 cup asparagus, chopped
1 clove garlic, minced
1 tsp. ginger, minced
1/2 tsp. red pepper flakes
1 Tbsp. organic teriyaki sauce
1 tsp. cilantro, chopped
1 tbsp. basil, chopped
non-stick cooking spray

Preparation: Cook rice. Spray a skillet with non-stick spray and heat on medium-low. When hot, add broccoli, mushrooms, onions, and asparagus. Cook for 3 to 4 minutes, stirring constantly. Add garlic, ginger, red pepper flakes, and teriyaki sauce and stir constantly for another minute. Combine cooked rice and vegetables in a bowl and top with basil and cilantro.

Makes 1 Serving
Nutritional Value: 212 calories; 10.3 g protein; 46 g carbs; 0.9 g fat; 7.9 g fiber; 285.5 mg sodium
Notes: Replacing any of the vegetables in this recipe with others such as carrots, zucchini, or bell peppers will not greatly change the nutritional value.

Diva Tuna Mixture

12 oz. solid white albacore tuna (canned in water or fresh),
2 Tbsp. mayonnaise
1/2 cup white onion, diced
1 1/2 cup celery, diced
1 kosher pickle, diced
1 tsp. lemon juice

Preparation: Thoroughly rinse tuna if using canned. In a bowl, mix together the tuna and mayonnaise. Add diced onions, celery, pickle, and lemon juice. Mix until all ingredients are well combined.

Makes 3 to 4 Servings — Recommended Serving Size: 3/4 cup
Nutritional Value Per Serving: 216.7 calories; 32.5 g protein; 3.7 g carbs; 7.7 g fat;
0.5 g fiber; 467 mg sodium
Notes: To reduce 100 mg of sodium per serving, eliminate the pickle and add a cucumber instead. To cut the fat in half, use low-fat mayonnaise. To add more fiber, add 1/4 cup chickpeas to the top. This is a great recipe to use as a spread, as part of a salad, and in a sandwich.

Soups, Salads & Sides

Diva Spicy Chicken Soup

1/2 cup brown rice
3 oz. cubed chicken breast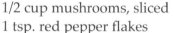
1/2 cup mushrooms, sliced
1 tsp. red pepper flakes
1 clove garlic, chopped
1 tsp. ginger, chopped
1 cup organic low-sodium beef broth
1 tsp. cilantro, chopped
2 Tbsp. green onions, chopped
non-stick cooking spray

Preparation: Cook brown rice. Spray a pot with non-stick spray and cook chicken on medium heat until almost cooked through. Then add mushrooms, red pepper flakes, garlic, and ginger and stir constantly about 2 minutes. Add beef broth and bring to a boil; make sure chicken is thoroughly cooked. Add cooked brown rice, cilantro and green onions; then serve.

Makes 1 Serving
Nutritional Value: 284 calories; 31.5 g protein; 28.8 g carbs; 4.3 g fat; 3.9 g fiber; 203 mg sodium

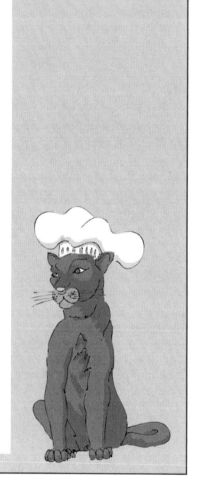

Diva No-Fat Soup in 30 Minutes

4 cups gluten-free vegetable broth
2 cups carrots, diced
8 garlic cloves, finely minced
3 Tbsp. shallots, finely minced
1 Tbsp. black pepper
1 Tbsp. oregano
1 cup white onion, diced
1 cup celery, diced
1 cup broccoli, diced

Preparation: In a pot combine and cook broth, carrots, garlic, shallots, black pepper, and oregano on medium heat for about 5 minutes. Add the onion and celery and continue cooking for another 2 minutes. Add the broccoli and cook for 2 minutes more. Reduce the heat to low and let simmer another 5 minutes.

Makes 3 Servings — Recommended Serving Size: 2 cups
Nutritional Value Per Serving: 110.9 calories; 5.5 g protein; 21.1 g carbs; 0.5 g fat; 6.1 g fiber; 418 mg sodium
Notes: Use different flavored broths to change the taste of this recipe. To reduce sodium level, use low-sodium broth.

Diva Onion Soup

1/2 Tbsp. olive oil
1 medium sweet onion, sliced
2 cups organic low-sodium beef broth
1 tsp. dried basil
1 Tbsp. Parmesan cheese, grated
black pepper

Preparation: Heat a pot on medium-low with the olive oil. Add onions and stir constantly; cook until softened, between 5 and 8 minutes. Add beef broth and basil and bring to a boil. Ladle soup into a bowl and top with Parmesan cheese and black pepper.

Makes 1 large serving
Nutritional Value: 172.5 calories; 8 g protein;
16.2 g carbs; 8.3 g fat; 3 g fiber; 230 mg sodium
Notes: To make this meal "non-beef" use vegetable broth.

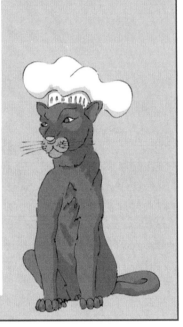

Diva Potato Salad

3 small red potatoes, cut in half
1 hard-boiled egg white, chopped
6 kalamata olives, chopped
1 Tbsp. capers, rinsed
1 Tbsp. red onion, chopped
1 Tbsp. green onion, chopped
1 Tbsp. reduced-fat light mayonnaise
1 Tbsp. yellow mustard
1 Tbsp. red wine vinegar
black pepper

Preparation: In a small saucepan, boil potatoes in water for about 10 minutes or until tender. Strain and rinse with cold water. When cool to touch, dice the potatoes into small squares and place into a mixing bowl. Add the chopped egg, olives, capers, and red and green onions to the potatoes. In a cup, mix together mayonnaise, mustard, and vinegar until well blended. Add wet mixture to potatoes and toss well. Add black pepper to taste.

Makes 2 Servings — Recommended Serving Size: half of the potato salad
Nutritional Value Per Serving: 248.3 calories; 7.2 g protein; 42.8 g carbs; 6.2 g fat;
4.1 g fiber; 369.5 mg sodium

Diva Spinach Salad

1 hard-boiled egg, chopped
3 cups baby spinach
1/2 cup mushrooms, sliced
2 Tbsp. light Italian dressing

Preparation: Combine all ingredients in a bowl and serve.

Makes 1 Serving
Nutritional Value: 140.5 calories; 9.3 g protein; 8.6 g carbs; 7.3 g fat;
2.5 g fiber; 479 mg sodium

Diva Bean Taco Salad

3 cups shredded romaine lettuce, shredded
1/2 cup kidney beans
6 black olives, chopped
1 Tbsp. cilantro, chopped
2 Tbsp. green onion, chopped
1 tomato, chopped
1/4 cup avocado, cubed
2 Tbsp. low fat Italian dressing

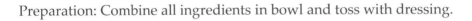

Preparation: Combine all ingredients in bowl and toss with dressing.

Makes 1 Serving
Nutritional Value: 273 calories; 12.5 g protein; 38 g carbs; 9.6 g fat;
10 g fiber; 428 mg sodium

Diva Colorful Raw Salad

1 cup cucumber, chopped
1 cup orange (or yellow) bell pepper, chopped
1/3 cup carrots, shredded
1/2 cup radishes, chopped
1/2 cup scallions, chopped
1/2 cup bean sprouts

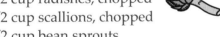

Preparation: Mix all ingredients in large bowl and enjoy!

Makes 4 to 5 Servings — Recommended Serving Size: 1 to 1 1/4 cup
Nutritional Value Per Serving: 50.7 calories; 2 g protein; 10 g carbs; 0.3 g fat;
3.3 g fiber; 21.3 mg sodium
Notes: You can add your favorite low-fat, low-sugar, no trans-fat dressing, but it will
change the nutritional value somewhat.

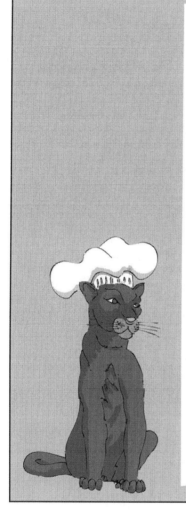

Diva Beet and Chicken Salad

1 beet, cooked, cooled and chopped
3 oz. chicken breast (from a rotisserie chicken), chopped or shredded
2 cups organic spring mix salad
1/3 cup carrots, shredded
1/3 cup peas, cooked and cooled
1 tomato, chopped
1 Tbsp. Balsamic vinaigrette dressing

Preparation: Place beet in small saucepan and boil for about 20 minutes or until *al dente*. Set aside and let cool slightly. While the beet is cooking, carve out the breast from your rotisserie chicken, cut into small pieces and set aside. Mix together spring mix, carrots, peas, and tomatoes. Add the beet and chicken (cold or warm). Toss with Balsamic vinaigrette.

Makes 1 Serving
Nutritional Value: 360 calories; 33.2 g protein; 31.5 g carbs; 9.5 g fat; 8.3 g fiber; 355 mg sodium

Diva Fresh Avocado Salsa

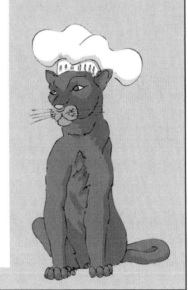

3 Roma tomatoes, diced
1/2 red onion, chopped
7 radish balls, chopped
1/4 cup green onions, chopped
1 Serrano chili pepper (or less if you can't handle
the heat)
2 avocados, diced
1/3 cup cilantro, chopped
juice of 1 lime
1 Tbsp. olive oil

Preparation: Mix together the first 7 ingredients
in a large bowl. Add the olive oil and then add
the lime juice.

Makes 7 Servings —
Recommended Serving Size: 1/2 to 3/4 cup
Nutritional Value Per Serving: 133 calories;
1.6 g protein; 10 g carbs; 10 g fat;
4.4 g fiber; 11.6 mg sodium

Diva Fresh Salsa

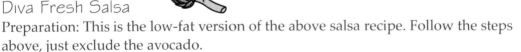

Preparation: This is the low-fat version of the above salsa recipe. Follow the steps
above, just exclude the avocado.

Makes 7 Servings — Recommended Serving Size: 1/4 to 1/2 cup
Nutritional Value Per Serving: 41.4 calories; 0.5 g protein; 5.3 g carbs; 2.4 g fat;
0.6 g fiber; 1.6 mg sodium

Supper

Diva Stove-top Halibut

4 oz. fresh Alaskan halibut
pinch of sea salt
1 tsp. rosemary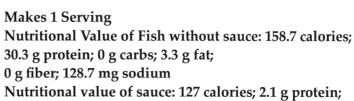
1 lemon, cut in half
1 shallot, finely chopped (1/3 cup)
1/2 Tbsp. olive oil
2 Tbsp. white wine (or other cooking wine)
non-stick cooking spray

Preparation: Season halibut with a pinch of sea salt and rosemary. Spray a skillet with non-stick cooking spray and heat on high. Reduce heat to medium and cook halibut for 3 minutes on each side. Squeeze juice of half the lemon over fish frequently to keep fish and pan moist. Reduce heat to low, cover skillet with a lid, and let cook 5 to 8 minutes on each side until done, or desired texture is reached.

In a separate skillet, sauté shallots in olive oil on medium heat for about 2 minutes. Add wine and juice of other lemon half. Reduce heat to low and let simmer for about 2 more minutes.

Place cooked fish on a plate and cover with the sauce.

Makes 1 Serving
Nutritional Value of Fish without sauce: 158.7 calories; 30.3 g protein; 0 g carbs; 3.3 g fat; 0 g fiber; 128.7 mg sodium
Nutritional value of sauce: 127 calories; 2.1 g protein; 13.9 g carbs; 7 g fat; 1.6 g fiber; 2 mg sodium

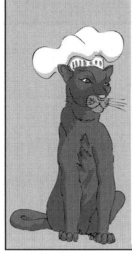

Diva Garlic Pepper Veggie Sauté

1/2 cup garlic, minced (about 1 whole head)
1 tsp. olive oil
7 mushrooms, quartered
1 red bell pepper, sliced
1 white onion, sliced
3 cups bean sprouts
1 tsp. black pepper

Preparation: In a skillet, sauté garlic in olive oil on medium heat for 1 to 2 minutes. Add all the veggies and black pepper. Cook until *al dente*, about 2 minutes.

Makes 2 Servings — Recommended Serving Size: 1 1/2 cups
Nutritional value Per Serving: 164 calories; 9.2 g protein; 28.2 g carbs; 3.1 g fat; 6.1 g fiber; 37.5 mg sodium
Notes: This recipe is for the garlic lover; if you prefer, use less garlic.

Diva Chicken Veggie Stir-Fry

3 oz. chicken breast, cut into bite-size pieces
1/2 cup broccoli, chopped
1/2 cup sliced mushrooms, sliced
1/2 cup yellow onions, chopped
1/2 cup asparagus, chopped
1 clove garlic, minced
1 tsp. ginger, minced
1/2 tsp. red pepper flakes
1 Tbsp. organic (gluten-free) teriyaki sauce
1 Tbsp. basil, chopped
1 tsp. cilantro, chopped
non-stick cooking spray

Preparation: Heat a skillet on medium-low and spray with non-stick spray. When hot, add chicken, broccoli, mushrooms, onions, and asparagus. Cook for 3 to 4 minutes, stirring constantly until chicken is cooked through. Add garlic, ginger, red pepper flakes, and teriyaki sauce and stir constantly for another minute. Transfer chicken and veggies to a bowl and top with basil and cilantro.

Makes 1 Serving
Nutritional Value: 246.5 calories; 34.5 g protein; 23.6 g carbs; 3.1 g fat;
6.3 g fiber; 334.5 mg sodium
Notes: Replacing any of the vegetables in this recipe for others (like eggplant, cauliflower, green beans or cabbage) will not greatly change the nutritional value.

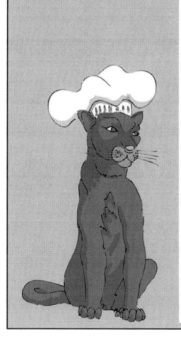

Diva Turkey Tacos

1/2 lb. lean ground turkey
1/2 tsp. red crushed chili pepper
1/4 tsp. peppercorn mélange
1/4 tsp. roasted garlic–sea salt blend
3 sprouted corn tortillas, warmed
non-stick cooking spray

Preparation: Spray a skillet with non-stick spray and start cooking ground turkey on medium heat. When halfway cooked, add chili pepper, peppercorns, and roasted garlic–sea salt blend. Constantly stirring, continue cooking another 5 minutes or until done. Spoon 1/3 of turkey meat onto one warm sprouted corn tortilla.

Makes 3 Servings —
Recommended Serving Size: 1 taco
Nutritional Value Per Serving 160 calories;
16.5 g protein; 11.5 g carbs; 5.5 g fat;
1.5 g fiber; 221.9 mg sodium
Notes: Topping the tacos with cilantro, onions, lettuce, and tomatoes adds few calories and lots of good nutrients. A handful of kidney, pinto, or black beans adds fiber.
Topping with 1/4 avocado or light cheese adds about another 7 grams of fat. Try to choose one or the other—not both (the avocado is a healthier choice).

Diva Vegetarian Tostada

1/2 cup organic refried pinto beans
2 flax and soy corn thins
1 cup loose-leaf lettuce
1 Tbsp. black olives, chopped
1/4 cup avocado, cubed
1/2 cup tomatoes, chopped

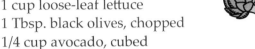

Preparation: Heat the beans in a pot on medium until warmed. Spread heated beans on both corn thins and decorate with the rest of your toppings.

Makes 1 Serving: 2 Tostadas
Nutritional Value: 228 calories; 10 g protein; 38.2 g carbs; 7.6 g fat;
12.9 g fiber; 287 mg sodium

Diva Chicken Fajitas

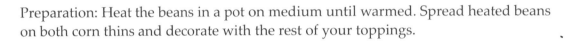

3 oz. chicken breast, cut in strips
1/2 cup green or red bell peppers, cut in strips
1/2 cup onions, sliced
dash of Italian seasoning
black pepper to taste
2 organic sprouted corn tortillas
1 Tbsp. fresh cilantro
2 Tbsp. organic salsa
non-stick cooking spray

Preparation: Spray a skillet with non-stick spray and heat on medium. Add chicken, peppers, onions, Italian seasoning, and black pepper, and constantly stir until the chicken is cooked through. Divide chicken and veggies on top of warmed tortillas; add cilantro and salsa.

Makes 1 Serving
Nutritional Value: 316 calories; 32.1 g protein; 37.1 g carbs; 4.3 g fat;
6.1 g fiber; 204 mg sodium

Diva Teriyaki Turkey Patty
1/2 lb. lean ground turkey
2 Tbsp. low-sodium, low-sugar, gluten-free teriyaki sauce
non-stick cooking spray

Preparation: In a ceramic or glass bowl, mix together ground turkey and teriyaki sauce. Marinate in the refrigerator all day. When ready to cook, form meat into two patties. Spray a skillet with non-stick spray and cook patties on medium heat until cooked through.

Makes 2 Servings — Recommended Serving Size: 1 patty
Nutritional Value: 185 calories; 22 g protein; 7 g carbs; 7 g fat;
0 g fiber; 380 mg sodium
Notes: Serve this with a large salad to make sure you get fiber in this meal.

Diva Special No-Bun Turkey Feta Burger

3 oz. lean ground turkey
1 tsp. olive oil
1 clove garlic, chopped
1 Tbsp. shallot, chopped
10 mushrooms, sliced
1 Tbsp. feta cheese
non-stick cooking spray

Preparation: First, form the turkey meat into a patty. Spray a skillet with non-stick spray and cook patty on medium heat until cooked through. While your turkey patty is cooking, heat olive oil in another skillet on medium and sauté garlic and shallots for about 2 minutes. Add the mushrooms and cook 4 to 5 minutes longer or until mushrooms are *al dente*. Transfer cooked turkey patty to a plate and top with mushroom mixture and feta cheese.

Makes 1 Serving
Nutritional Value: 305 calories; 38.5 g protein; 9.9 g carbs; 15.3 g fat; 2.3 g fiber; 406 mg sodium
Notes: To make this recipe a non-dairy meal, skip the cheese. This will also lower the fat by about 5 grams or so. You can also use kosher, lean ground beef once in a while to make this dish. Just skip the cheese to keep the fat grams in check.

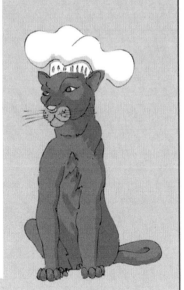

Alternatives to Any Meal

Diva Protein Shake

2 scoops of quality protein powder
1/4 cup plain low fat yogurt
1/2 banana
1/4 cup mixed berries (frozen or fresh)
1/4 cup water

Preparation: Combine first 4 ingredients in a blender or Magic Bullet, add water and mix until well blended.

Makes 1 Shake
Nutritional Value: 334.5 calories; 24 g protein; 58 g carbs; 1.6 g fat;
10 g fiber; 170 mg sodium
Nutritional Value of 1 Tbsp. flaxseeds: 48 calories; 2 g protein; 3.3 g carbs; 3.3 g fat;
2.7 g fiber; 3.4 mg sodium
Notes: You can use juice instead of water. For a lower-calorie, lower-protein, and lower-carbohydrate shake, use only 1 scoop of protein powder. You can add flaxseeds to add more nutritional value (including omega-3 fatty acids, fiber, and magnesium, plus the added benefits to your heart, digestion, and protections against certain cancers). You can substitute whatever fruit you like.

Diva High-Fiber Smoothie

1 cup strawberries (frozen or fresh)
1 cup mixed berries (frozen or fresh)
1/2 cup soy milk

Preparation: Mix all ingredients in a blender until smooth.

Makes 1 Smoothie
Nutritional Value: 175 calories; 5.4 g protein; 35.5 g carbs; 2.6 g fat;
13.4 g fiber; 61.4 mg sodium

Diva Veggie Drink

1 beet
2 carrots
1 cup broccoli

Preparation: Mix all ingredients in a juicer and enjoy!

Makes 1 Drink
Nutritional Value: 200 calories; 8.8 g protein; 39.6 g carbs; 0.8 g fat;
12 g fiber; 220 mg sodium

Diva Lunch Box Meals

Diva LB Meal #1

3 oz. leftover grilled chicken breast
1 sliced apple with 1 Tbsp. low-fat peanut butter
1/2 cup sliced cucumber and 1/2 cup shredded carrot salad with 1
Tbsp. white wine vinegar

Makes 1 Lunch
Nutritional Value: 352 calories; 31.6 g protein; 36.6 g carbs; 9.4 g fat;
7.2 g fiber; 204 mg sodium

Diva LB Meal #2

1 hard-boiled egg
1 cup broccoli with 1 cup cauliflower dipped in
2 Tbsp. low-fat ranch dressing
1 large banana
Notes: Change the dressing to make a non-dairy meal.

Makes 1 Lunch
Nutritional Value: 295 calories; 12.8 g protein; 45.9 g carbs; 7.8 g fat;
8 g fiber; 413 mg sodium

Diva LB Meal #3
1/2 cup 2% low-fat cottage cheese
1 cup diced cantaloupe
1 cup pre-boiled green peas

Makes 1 Lunch
Nutritional Value: 295 calories; 25.6 g protein; 43.5 g carbs; 2.9 g fat; 10.4 g fiber; 491.8 mg sodium

Diva LB Meal #4
3 oz. leftover turkey breast
6 oz. organic fat-free yogurt
1 cup fresh blueberries

Makes 1 Lunch
Nutritional Value: 336 calories; 32.5 g protein; 46 g carbs; 3.2 g fat; 5.5 g fiber; 161 mg sodium

Diva LB Meal #5
I piece string cheese
4 oz. container organic applesauce
1 ear leftover corn on the cob

Makes 1 Lunch
Nutritional Value: 237 calories; 10 g protein; 37 g carbs; 7.1 g fat; 4.4 g fiber; 224 mg sodium

Diva LB Meal #6
1/4 cup fresh trail mix, no salt
1 large orange

Makes 1 Lunch
Nutritional Value: 191.6 calories; 5.2 g protein; 28.4 g carbs; 9.2 g fat; 5.1 g fiber; 15 mg sodium

MY DIVA DIET Food Preparation, Cooking, and Meal Planning Guide: 52 Tips

This section of MY DIVA DIET is not meant to be a cookbook, but rather it serves as a quick guide to help get you in the kitchen to prepare healthy and fit meals. For a complete and healthy guide to cooking, try *The World's Healthiest Foods* by George Mateljan *www.worldshealthiestfoods.com*.

> There are many cookbooks on the market today—just pick the ones that make good health a top priority. Then we can take any healthy recipe and make it fit (for fat reduction).

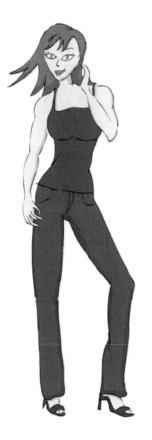

Whether you are the chef at home or someone else is doing the cooking, these tips help create healthy, fit foods that taste great. You can also cross-reference this guide with the MY DIVA DIET Restaurant Eating Guide to ensure all your cooking is appropriate for fat loss and wellness (this means physical well-being, achieved through a good diet and exercise).

Cooking Tips

#1.　　Avoid microwave cooking, if possible, because it destroys the enzymes in foods.

#2.　　Cooking can be quick and healthy if you are prepared. Stock your kitchen with the right tools for cooking.

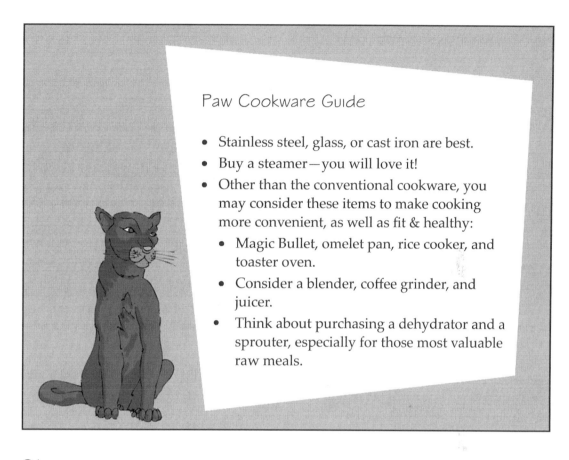

Paw Cookware Guide

- Stainless steel, glass, or cast iron are best.
- Buy a steamer—you will love it!
- Other than the conventional cookware, you may consider these items to make cooking more convenient, as well as fit & healthy:
  - Magic Bullet, omelet pan, rice cooker, and toaster oven.
  - Consider a blender, coffee grinder, and juicer.
  - Think about purchasing a dehydrator and a sprouter, especially for those most valuable raw meals.

Oils

#3. Cooking without oil is a good idea for two reasons: oil can be damaged in the heating process, and oil adds more fat to a dish.

#4. Some oil is more resistant to heat than others. In fact, depending on the temperature and the type of oil used, it can even become harmful. When cooking with oil, it is best to use a high-oleic version of sunflower or safflower oils. Olive oil (extra-virgin) is too sensitive for cooking at high temperatures, but can be used when cooking at low to medium temperatures.

#5. It's okay to use non-stick cooking sprays. Make sure they do not contain alcohol and other harmful ingredients. Check that the oils used are unsaturated (like sunflower, safflower, olive, and canola). A good product is Trader Joe's Extra-Virgin Italian Olive Oil Spray.

#6. Olive oil is great on salads and in sauces. It's best to use organic, cold-pressed, extra-virgin olive oil.

Herbs, Spices and Other Seasonings

#7. For the many health benefits, few calories, and great flavor, you can't ignore the value of using herbs, spices, and vegetables in your cooking. There are many to choose from, such as garlic, onions, leeks, basil, pepper, oregano, sage, cinnamon, turmeric, rosemary, black pepper, coriander, parsley, thyme, dill weed, and others. Fruit is another way to add flavor and nutrients to your dishes.

#8. Keep many herbs and spices—such as fresh basil, cilantro, oregano, and pepper— readily available. You never know when you will need them for a specific dish.

#9. It is best to purchase herbs and spices fresh, but if they are not, make sure they are untainted. Be leery of herbs and spices that have been packaged—especially the ones that are mixed with other ingredients and additives that are not beneficial to health.

#10. Salt is okay to use, but do not drown the flavor of your foods. It is best to use sea salt or kosher salt—not refined table salt.

#11. You don't really need to cook with sugar at all, in any circumstance. For baking, consider a pure high-quality honey or agave nectar.

#12. When using beef or chicken broth, use an organic, low-sodium, gluten-free product.

Beef, Poultry, Fish and Eggs

#13. Beef, poultry and fish should be baked, broiled, or grilled—never breaded or deep-fried. You can stir-fry your meats and poultry, but watch the amount of oil you use. Try poaching your fish; it is an easy and mild way to prepare fish.

#14. Eggs and egg whites can be scrambled or made omelet-style. Hard-boiled and poached are other great options.

Whole Grains

#15. Whole grains are easy to prepare (use a rice cooker for perfect rice). Oats, quinoa, buckwheat, and other whole grains are easy to prepare as well, and some can be prepared using your rice cooker.

#16. Whole grains can be used raw or cooked in any recipes—in soups, stews, salads, and for baking, and they are a great substitute for bread crumbs.

#17. Whole grains are enjoyable to use as a side dish to any meal.

#18. Whole grains taste superior alone. You don't need to add anything when cooking or serving. But, if you must, here are some ideas that add flavor without adding junk.

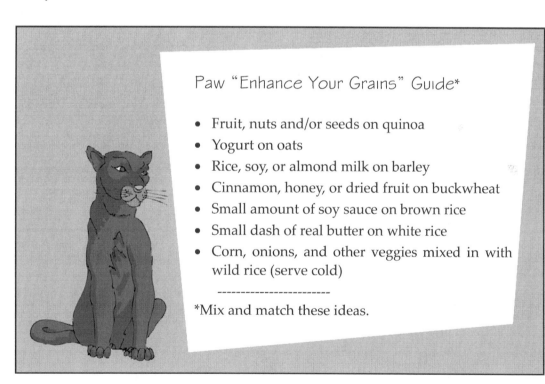

Paw "Enhance Your Grains" Guide*

- Fruit, nuts and/or seeds on quinoa
- Yogurt on oats
- Rice, soy, or almond milk on barley
- Cinnamon, honey, or dried fruit on buckwheat
- Small amount of soy sauce on brown rice
- Small dash of real butter on white rice
- Corn, onions, and other veggies mixed in with wild rice (serve cold)

----

*Mix and match these ideas.

Potatoes and Yams
#19. Bake or boil your potatoes and yams. You can eat the skin too!

#20. Baked potatoes have a fine flavor, but you may want a little extra. Skip the traditional way of topping your baked potato (butter, sour cream, and bacon) because this packs way too many calories, contains bad foods, and masks the potato's natural flavor. Try the MY DIVA DIET way of eating a potato—one that keeps it a low calorie, high nutrient meal that tastes good.

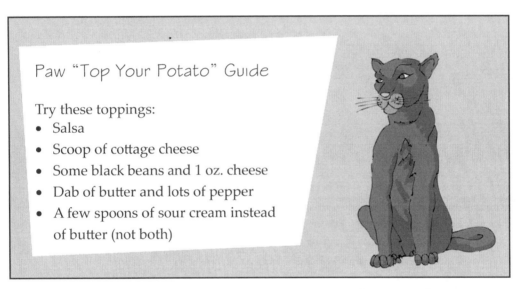

Paw "Top Your Potato" Guide

Try these toppings:
- Salsa
- Scoop of cottage cheese
- Some black beans and 1 oz. cheese
- Dab of butter and lots of pepper
- A few spoons of sour cream instead
  of butter (not both)

#21. Eat a cooked yam like an apple. This is a great on-the-go snack.

#22. Yams are best left alone with their sweet flavor, but try a few dashes of cinnamon and/or or a dab of real butter.

Legume, Nuts and Seeds
#23. Try germinating and/or sprouting your own legumes, nuts, and seeds. That way you get the entire raw benefit and avoid any man-manipulated food problems.

#24. Legumes, nuts, and seeds are enjoyable alone, as a snack, side dish, and in many recipes. They are a nice addition to baking, especially when making your own bread or other baked goods.

#25. Legumes, nuts, and seeds should be used often as they are a good source of protein and most are high in fiber. See how you can add more of these to your diet below.

Paw "Use Your Legumes, Nuts, and Seeds Often" Guide

Legumes
Use in these ways:
- With other vegetables to make a bean soup
- In soups and salads
- To top a salad
- In wraps and sandwiches
- In tacos and burritos
- With other veggies to make a great high-fiber meal
- To make dips and spreads (like bean dip and hummus)

Nuts and Seeds
Use in these ways:
- To top a salad or soup (sunflower seeds or walnuts)
- To top any veggie dish
- To use as an ingredient in a dish, such as cashew chicken (cashews, sesame and pumpkin seeds)
- With whole grains as a topping or addition (almonds)
- As a spread (almond, peanut, and cashew butter)
- In homemade dressings (flaxseed and almonds)
- In protein shakes or smoothies (flaxseed)
- To mix with dried fruit to make a healthy trail mix

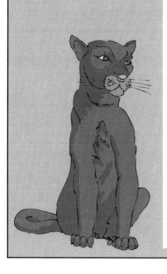

Vegetables

#26. Raw vegetables are best. But if you need to cook your veggies, they should be baked, grilled, roasted, or steamed. Stir-fried and sautéed are other ways to prepare veggies; just watch the amount of oil used.

#27. When you cook your veggies, make sure to do it quickly. Do not overcook your vegetables—nutrients get damaged and flavor is lost.

#28. Better to have all foods *al dente* than overcooked (exceptions are eggs, meats, and fish).

#29. Your veggies have their own wonderful flavors; don't drown them with sauces, butter, oils, or salt.

Salads

#30. Be creative with your salads and choose a variety of vegetables. Who said that green lettuce is the only way to make a salad? Use colors!

#31. Try adding other veggies to your salad (like raw celery and cooled asparagus) to add more nutrients and fiber.

#32. Add some legumes, nuts, and seeds (like chickpeas, peas, almonds, and sunflower seeds) to your salad to add crunch and more protein and fiber.

#33. Try chopping your salad ingredients into smaller sizes to create a different texture from your average salad.

#34. When making a salad, make a little extra for the next day. To prevent soggy veggies, don't add dressing to the entire salad. These extra veggies will be great for next-day, omelets, sandwiches, wraps, salads, or snacks.

#35. Make sure you don't drown your salad with dressing. Pepper is a great natural flavor enhancer for all salads and other dishes. Did you know peppercorns offer a digestive aid, provide an important antioxidant, have an antibiotic activity, and help with weight control?

#36. Try adding only Balsamic vinegar to your salad or veggies—it has barely any calories and is full of flavor.

Soups

#37. When making soup, it is best to make it broth-based. Cream soups require high-fat type products. Again, use a variety of vegetables, legumes, nuts, seeds, herbs, and spices.

#38. Always choose low-sodium and low-fat broth when making soup so that your bowl of soup does not contain your entire daily allowance of sodium milligrams and fat grams.

#39. When making soup, make a little extra for the next day's snack, lunch, or side-dish. You can even freeze single servings of leftover soup.

Cheese

#40. Be cautious when using cheese in your food preparation, in any recipe or as a topping. Cheese is high in calories and fat grams. Try using Parmesan, Romano, or feta cheese to add flavor without adding too many calories—a small amount goes a long way.

Canned Foods

#41. When using canned foods (like tuna, legumes, olives, etc.), choose low-sodium brands and make sure you rinse the contents thoroughly with water to eliminate as much sodium as possible. Even though products are labeled low-sodium, some are not low enough.

Sides

#42. Think about using fruit as a side dish, garnish, or dessert.

#43. Try whole grain or rice pasta and serve it as a side dish to control the serving size and amount of calories.

#44. For a low-carbohydrate meal, skip the pasta and just have some tomato sauce with turkey meatballs and a side salad.

#45. Try spaghetti squash with some marinara as a side dish. This is a great low-carbohydrate, high-nutrient idea.

Planning Ahead
#46. Make extra of whatever you're cooking for another meal.
- Make a few chicken breasts or turkey patties for the next day's lunch. Make a large bowl of veggies so you have food the next day for your breakfast omelet, snack, or salad.

#47. Keep a few hard-boiled eggs handy to use for a quick breakfast or snack.

#48. Always have a freshly baked chicken or turkey on hand as some pure protein ready to add to your salad, soup, sandwich, or wrap. This is even good for your next-day lunch item.

#49. When you know you are going to be away from home for more than three hours try to:
- Eat before you go.
- Carry snack items with you.
- Know where to get healthy, fit foods.
- Know where to get clean and pure smoothies and protein shakes.

Extras
#50. Try some of the "Spice Up Your Meals" products as ingredients or additions to your recipes and meals. These give lots of spice without too many calories, too much sodium, and unneeded sugar or white flour.

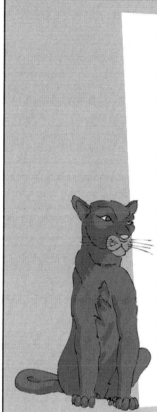

Paw "Spice Up Your Meals" Guide

To add flavor and variety to your dishes, try these wholesome additions:
- Applesauce (sugar-free)
- Balsamic vinegar
- Chickpeas and/or kidney beans
- Horseradish
- Mustard
- Olives and olive oil
- Light (low-sodium) soy sauce
- Light (low-sodium, low-sugar, and gluten-free) teriyaki sauce
- Low-sodium, low-fat, and gluten-free broth
- No-sugar marinara sauce
- Salsa and healthy hot sauce
- Sesame, sunflower seeds, flaxseeds, and many other fruits, veggies, herbs, and spices

See our more complete Herbs and Spices section in PART SEVEN for great ways to add flavor, nutrients, and medicinal usage for a given meal or recipes—without the extra calories!

#51. Last but not least, keep your refrigerator clean.

#52. If you don't cook, see the MY DIVA DIET Restaurant Eating Guide in PART SIX.

Diva Smart Diet Cheat Sheet
Phase One—Diva Reduction

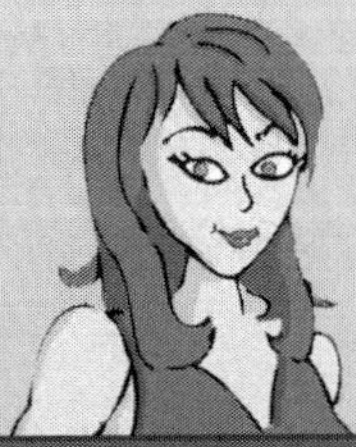

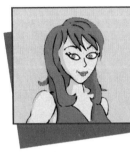

"When it comes to cheating—keep it simple and safe, and the fewer ingredients the better! Also keep your cheats to once per week or less."

Paw "Smart Diet Cheats" Guide

* Only use once per week or less
  Keep to one serving or 50 to 200 calories
- The fewer ingredients the better
- Choose pure ingredients, always
- Choose natural, fresh, organic, and kosher foods when possible
- Choose wholesome foods (foods with nutritional value)
- Choose foods low in fat, sugar, and sodium
- Low- or non-fat dairy cheats are okay
- Choose foods low in saturated fats and cholesterol
- Gluten-free foods are a good idea
- Flours made from wheat, potato, masa, spelt, and rye are okay
- Certain white-flour products are okay on occasion, like no-salt sourdough pretzels, sourdough bread, and white pasta.

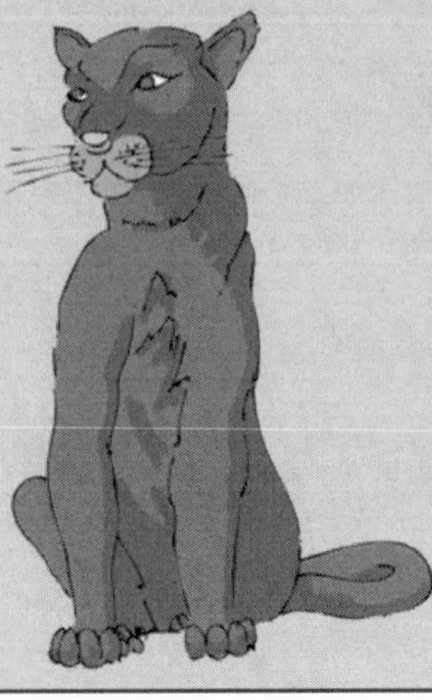

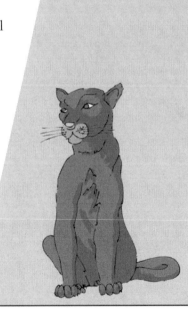

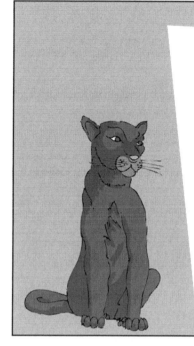

Paw "Smart Diet Cheats" Guide
Continued....

- Healthy cereals would be another way to cheat safely (just don't eat the whole box!).
- Dark chocolate is always a good cheat choice, as are fudgsicles, puddings and popcicles.
- Don't be tempted to choose items that contain artificial ingredients, hydrogenated oils, high-fructose corn syrup, sodium nitrate, and other harmful preservatives and additives.

Smart Diet Cheats

MY DIVA DIET cheats for dieting are allowed within the guidelines above, so enjoy!

- These simple and safe cheat ideas meet the Paw "Smart Diet Cheats" Guide.
- Ideas are gluten-free.
- Some have flour and some have dairy.
- Some have higher amounts of sugar, as most treats do, unless you are into salty foods.
- Some contain sodium.
- Items are listed by product name and serving size, followed by the nutrition facts.
- If you do your own research, you can find other cheats that fit this criteria and the Paw Guide above.

Cold & Creamy

•Kozy Shack Chocolate Pudding: Serving size: 1/2 cup
140 calories; 4 g protein; 24 g carbs; 3 g fat; 1 g fiber; 19 g sugar; 140 mg sodium

•FudgStix Lite: Serving size: 1 bar
90 calories; 3 g protein; 18 g carbs; 0.5 g fat; 1 g fiber; 9 g sugar; 45 mg sodium

•FruitStix Creamy Coconut: Serving size: 1 bar
110 calories; 2 g protein; 18 g carbs; 4 g fat; 0 g fiber; 8 g sugar; 3 mg sodium

•FruitStix Creamy Banana Low-Fat: Serving size: 1 bar
90 calories; 1 g protein; 17 g carbs; 2 g fat; 0 g fiber; 9 g sugar; 30 mg sodium

•Julie's Organic Sorbet (blackberry): Serving size 1 bar
60 calories; 0 g protein; 16 g carbs; 0 g fat; 0 g fiber; 14 g sugar; 20 mg sodium

•Dreyer's Vanilla Fat-Free Yogurt: Serving size 1/2 cup
90 calories; 3 g protein; 20 g carbs; 0 g fat; 0 g fiber; 14 g sugar; 45 mg sodium

•Dreyer's Swiss Orange Sherbet: Serving size: 1/2 cup
150 calories; 1 g protein; 30 g carbs; 3 g fat; 0 g fiber; 25 g sugar; 40 mg sodium

•Breyers All-Natural Vanilla Ice Cream: Serving size: 1/2 cup
140 calories; 3 g protein; 15 g carbs; 7 g fat; 0 g fiber; 15 g sugar; 40 mg sodium

•Yoplait Chocolate Mousse Whips: Serving size: 1 container
160 calories; 5 g protein; 26 g carbs; 4 g fat; 0 g fiber; 23 g sugar; 105 mg sodium

•Yoplait Raspberry Cheesecake Thick & Creamy: Serving size: 6 oz.
190 calories; 7 g protein; 32 g carbs; 3.5 g fat; 0 g fiber; 28 g sugar; 100 mg sodium

Chocolate
•Xocai Chocolate Nuggets: Serving size: 12g
70 calories; 1 g protein; 6 g carbs; 5 g fat; 1 g fiber; 3 g sugar; 10 mg sodium

•Dove Dark Bar: Serving size: 12g
70 calories; 1 g protein; 7 g carbs; 4 g fat; 0 g fiber; 7 g sugar; 8 mg sodium

•CocoaVia Chocolate-Covered Almonds: Serving size: 1 pack (best to eat only half)
140 calories; 3 g protein; 12 g carbs; 11 g fat; 3 g fiber; 8 g sugar; 0 mg sodium

Candy Type
•Yummy Earth Mixed Fruit Lollipops: Serving size: 3 lollipops
70 calories; 0 g protein; 17 g carbs; 0 g fat; 0 g fiber; 17 g sugar; 0 mg sodium

Cookies

•My-Deal Gluten-Free/Dairy-Free Ginger Snaps: Serving size: 5 cookies
140 calories; 2 g protein; 21 g carbs; 6 g fat; 1 g fiber; 12 g sugar; 85 mg sodium

•Sans Gluten-Free Vanilla-Flavored Wafer Cookies: Serving size: 4 wafers
160 calories; 1 g protein; 19 g carbs; 8 g fat; 3 g fiber; 14 g sugar; 25 mg sodium

•Barbara's Fig Bars – Wheat-Free: Serving size: 1 bar
60 calories; 1 g protein; 13 g carbs; 0 g fat; 1 g fiber; 8 g sugar; 25 mg sodium

Chips, Crackers & Crunch

•Pinnacle Gold Natural Gluten-Free Baked Potato Chips: Serving size: 1 oz.
110 calories; 2 g protein; 19 g carbs; 1.5 g fat; 2 g fiber; 2 g sugar; 160 mg sodium

•Lundberg Wasabi Rice Chips: Serving size: 1 oz.
140 calories; 2 g protein; 18 g carbs; 6 g fat; 1 g fiber; 1 g sugar; 210 mg sodium

•R.W. Garcia Lo's Tortilla Chips: Serving size: 1 oz.
140 calories; 6 g protein; 13 g carbs; 8 g fat; 4 g fiber; 0 g sugar; 50 mg sodium

•Edward & Son Vegetable Baked Brown Rice Snaps: Serving size: 8 crackers
60 calories; 1 g protein; 12 g carbs; 1 g fat; 1 g fiber; 1 g sugar; 40 mg sodium

•The Kitchen Table Bakers Gourmet Cheese Crisps: Serving size: 3 crackers
80 calories; 7 g protein; 1 g carbs; 6 g fat; 0 g fiber; 0 g sugar; 150 mg sodium

•Orville Redenbacher's Buttered Popcorn Mini Cakes: Serving size: 8 cakes
60 calories; 2 g protein; 12 g carbs; 1 g fat; 1 g fiber; 0 g sugar; 70 mg sodium

•Mrs. May's Naturals
Pumpkin Crunch: Serving
size: 6 pieces
98 calories; 9 g protein;
8 carbs; 11 g fat; 1 g fiber;
4 g sugar; 41 mg sodium

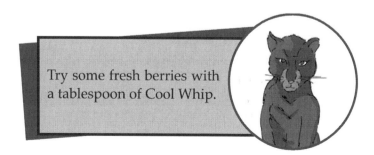

Try some fresh berries with a tablespoon of Cool Whip.

MY DIVA DIET Grocery Shopping Guide

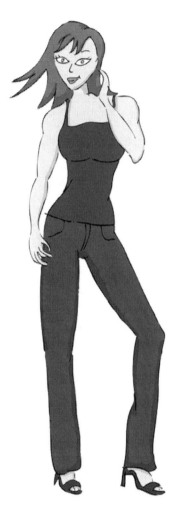

#1. If possible, try shopping at a natural or health food store. This helps you pick healthy, natural foods. These stores also give you a bigger selection of organic and kosher meats, fresh water fish, eggs from free-range vegetarian fed hens, organic dairy products, fresh organic fruits and vegetables. Great places to shop are Trader Joes (www.traderjoes.com) and Whole Food Markets (www.wholefoodsmarket.com).

#2. Know where your own local health-conscious grocery store is.

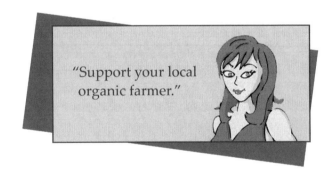

"Support your local organic farmer."

#3. Find your local organic farmer and/or farmers' market to get your fresh produce.

#4. Shop from the outside aisles in. The outside aisles have all the fresh produce, herbs, meats and fish, as well as dairy and other products that require refrigeration. These are where most of your "good foods" are.

#5. Do not go to the grocery store when you are hungry. This might cause you to break down and buy everything.

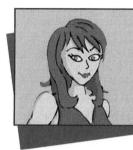

"Don't be fooled by all the products at a
health food store. Some are not as safe to
eat as real, wholesome, fresh foods are.
And you can gain weight from eating too
much—even from good foods!"

#6.   Make grocery shopping easier by making a list. This enables you to pick what you
need instead of items you don't. It is also more efficient to make a list, thus saving
time and money!

#7.   Use the MY DIVA DIET grocery shopping tools.

Paw Grocery Shopping Tools

- Diva Reduction Meal Options and Recipes
- Diva Smart Diet Cheat Sheet
- Paw Grocery Cart Check Guide
- Diva Reduction Good Food Choices At-a-Glance
- Diva Reduction Safe Cereal List
- Diva Food Test and Paw Label Guide

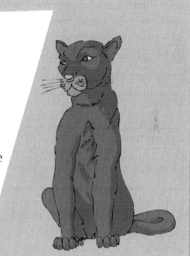

#8.   Take your own meal and recipe ideas with you.

#9.   Plan your meal ideas in advance so that you don't waste time or food.

#10. Resist the junk-food items!

#11. Make sure you buy your planned cheat items so you won't cheat on something you shouldn't.

#12. Skip the deli section unless it is a health food store and you know what is in the pre-made dishes. Exceptions are rotisserie chickens, fresh turkey breast, high-quality deli meats, and some salads.

#13. Always read labels when you are buying any food in a package.

#14. When you check out, do a quick glance at your basket.

#15. Final Tip: For more help on what foods to buy, see our name-brand list in MY DIVA DIET Resources and Recommendations at the end of this book.

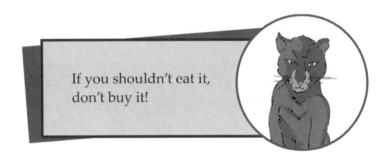

If you shouldn't eat it, don't buy it!

Paw Grocery Cart Check Guide

✓ Your grocery cart should be filled with fresh fruit and vegetables.

✓ While you were in the produce aisle, did you also remember your herbs and spices?

✓ Did you pick up some water and tea (or coffee)?

✓ Check for a few lean meats (like skinless chicken breasts and ground turkey).

✓ If it is a beef night, add some filet mignon to your cart.

✓ If it is a fish night, select some fresh wild salmon, halibut, or snapper.

✓ Add a few deli items (like baked chicken and fresh cuts of deli meat).

✓ Be sure your dairy products are low- or no-fat.

✓ Include a variety of legumes, nuts, seeds, and some almond or nut butter.

✓ Choose a few healthy plant protein products (like soy milk and hummus).

✓ Add a variety of whole grains (like quinoa, rice, buckwheat, and oats).

✓ Check for a few grain products (like mochi, rice cakes, sprouted corn tortillas, and safe cereals).

✓ Don't forget the olive oil and Balsamic vinegar.

✓ If you buy salad dressing, make sure it's low-fat, low-sodium, and sugar-free.

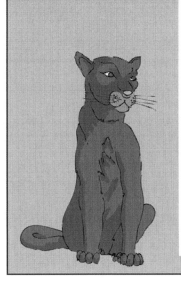

Paw Grocery Cart Check Guide
Continued....

✓ Do you have some Parmesan cheese and other good foods for flavor (like salsa and marinara)?
✓ You should have very few sauces—but you can add mustard and horseradish.
✓ Add some honey or agave nectar, a small container of fruit spread, and some applesauce.
✓ Add a few selections of dried fruit.
✓ Be sure you have very few canned or frozen foods—maybe some peas, chickpeas, and kidney beans. Or some tuna, corn, olives, and berries.
✓ Did you grab some smart diet cheats?
✓ Did you check the dates on packaged foods?
✓ Did you read the labels on your packaged foods before you dropped them into your cart?

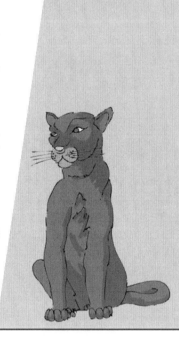

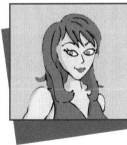

"Always choose natural, fresh, organic, and kosher foods. It may mean you spend a little more money and make more trips to the grocery store, but it also means fewer visits to the doctor's office."

Paw "Good Food Choices" Quick Guide

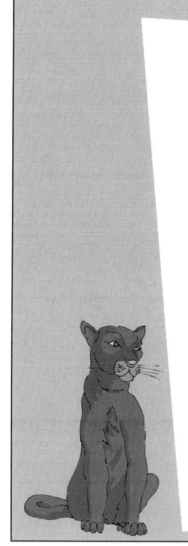

- Fresh-water fish (with fins and scales)
- Organic free-range and grass-fed animal meats (beef, poultry, turkey)
- Kosher meats
- Eggs from organic, free-range, vegetarian-fed hens
- Organic low- to no-fat dairy
- Fresh legumes
- Raw and unsalted nuts and seeds
- Plant protein products—clean and pure
- Organic whole grains
- Grain products—sprouted, stone ground (baked, never fried)
- Organic fresh fruits and vegetables
- Fresh and untainted herbs and spices
- Extra-virgin olive oil and other unrefined vegetable oils
- All-natural spreads, sauces, sweeteners, salad dressings, and dips.
- All-natural gluten-free smart diet cheats

PART SIX

Other Tools

Failure is impossible.
~ Susan B. Anthony

Diva Reduction Good Food Choices At-a-Glance
(with Nutritional Values)

Unless you are a nutritionist, food expert, or well-informed fitness professional making good food choices can be a confusing subject. Even experts sometimes disagree on what to eat. There are obvious choices of what not to eat, namely most packaged, processed, and man-made foods–especially the ones full of preservatives and additives. However, some packaged and man-made foods may be good to eat, and some may even be a smart diet cheat. As you do your own research on packaged and man-made foods you can add more of them to your diet. Just remember that when you consume more man-made foods, you are increasing your odds of making mistakes in your food choices.

We want to make your food choices easier by providing you with a readily available list of what MY DIVA DIET will have you eat during Phase One–Diva Reduction of the program and can be used in Phase Two–Diva Maintenance as well. This will aid you with your meal planning and ensure that you get all of the vitamins, minerals, fiber, antioxidants, phytochemicals, and other benefits that each food offers–plus you won't get bored. We could list what not to eat but that would require an entire book of foods! We are also providing you with the nutritional value of these foods rounded to the to the nearest tenth (keep in mind that calorie counters vary in their analysis).

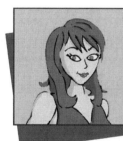

"Pure and wholesome foods (God/nature-made foods) will always be a staple in any diet, whether you want to lose fat, improve health, gain lean body mass, increase your fitness level, become an athlete, or even just maintain your current weight and health condition."

There are things that may change within the Five Factors, including amount of exercise, liquid consumption, total calories and nutriet ratio, as well as the frequency of diet cheating. Medical problems, allergies, and religious beliefs may also force you to give up certain "good foods".

Protein

Animal protein
Fish:
Choose clean, wild, fresh fish with scales and fins.

- Low-fat fish: cod, flounder, haddock, halibut, perch, Pollack, red snapper, sea bass, rainbow trout, and yellow fin tuna
- Fatty fish: freshwater bass, bluefish, mullet, orange roughy, and blue fin tuna
- High fat fish: herring, mackerel, pompano, salmon, and sardines

FOOD CHART

Fish (all 3 oz. fresh & cooked)	Calories	Protein (g)	Carbs (g)	Fat (g)
Bluefish	135	21.8	0	4.6
Cod	89	19.4	0	0.7
Flounder and Sole	99	20.5	0	1.3
Haddock	95	20.6	0	0.8
Halibut	119	22.7	0	2.5
Herring (Pacific)	213	17.9	0	15.1
Mackerel (Atlantic)	223	20.3	0	15.1
Mullet	128	21.1	0	4.1
Orange Roughy	76	16	0	0.8
Perch	100	20	0	2
Pompano	179	20.1	0	10.3
Salmon (Pacific)	184	23	0	9.3
Sea Bass	105	20	0	2.2
Snapper	109	22	0	1.5
Trout	128	22	0	3.7
Tuna	156	25	0	5.3
White Fish	92	20	0	0.8
Canned White Tuna (in water)	116	22.7	0	2.1

Poultry: Chicken and Turkey
Choose, lean kosher white poultry without the skin.
- Dark meat poultry on occasion
- Try poultry in a lean ground form

FOOD CHART

Poultry	Calories	Protein (g)	Carbs (g)	Fat (g)
Chicken (all 3 oz. chicken meat only)				
Breast	142	26.7	0	3.1
Drumsticks	151	24.9	0	5
Thighs	109	13.5	0	5.7
Turkey (all 3 oz. meat only)				
Dark meat	159	24.3	0	6.1
White meat	133	25.4	0	2.7
Ground turkey breast (4 oz.)	120	28	0	1.5

Note: These each contain 50 to 85 mg of cholesterol.

Beef:

Choose lean kosher beef, trim the fat and only eat once a month or less.

- Filet mignon, flank, top sirloin, extra lean ground beef, porterhouse, rib eye, shank, T-bone, etc.

FOOD CHART

Beef (all 3 oz. lean only- broiled, braised, or roasted)	Calories	Protein (g)	Carbs (g)	Fat (g)
Filet Mignon	179	24	0	8.5
Flank Steak	176	23	0	8.6
Ground Beef	218	21.6	0	13.9
Porterhouse Steak	185	23.9	0	9.2
Rib eye Steak	191	23.8	0	10
Shank Cross Cuts	171	28.6	0	5.4
Sirloin Steak	166	25.8	0	6.1
T-Bone Steak	182	23.9	0	8.8
Tip Round Steak	157	24.4	0	5.9
Top Loin Steak	176	24.3	0	8
Top Round Steak	153	26.9	0	4.2

Note: These each contain 60 to 80 mg of cholesterol.

Other meats like lamb, veal and duck:

Choose lean cuts and kosher.

- Should only be eaten only on special occasions

FOOD CHART

Other Meats	Calories	Protein (g)	Carbs (g)	Fat (g)
Lamb (all 3 oz. lean only-broiled or roasted)				
Foreshank	159	26.4	0	5
Rib Roast	197	22.2	0	11.3
Shank	153	23.9	0	5.7
Sirloin	173	24.1	0	7.8
Veal (all 3 oz. lean only-broiled, braised, or roasted)				
Ground	146	20.7	0	6.4
Loin	149	22.4	0	5.9
Sirloin	143	22.4	0	5.3
Duck (3 oz.) Broiled				
Breast Meat w/o skin	171	20	0	9.5

Note: These each contain 75 to 90 mg of cholesterol.

Whole eggs and egg whites:
Choose cage-free hens that are fed a 100% vegetarian diet.

FOOD CHART

Eggs	Calories	Protein (g)	Carbs (g)	Fat (g)	Fiber (g)	Sodium (mg)
Whole Egg (1)	75	6.3	0.6	5	0	70
Egg White (1)	17	3.6	0.2	0	0	55
Egg Yolk (1)	55	2.7	1	4.5	0	7
Hard Boiled (1 whole egg)	78	6.3	0.6	5.3	0	7
Hard Boiled (1 white)	17	3.6	0.2	0.1	0	55

Note: Egg yolks contain 213 mg of cholesterol while egg whites contain zero!

Other Meat Products—one choice:
Choose fresh deli cuts of chicken or turkey breast

FOOD CHART

Deli Meats	Calories	Protein (g)	Carbs (g)	Fat (g)	Fiber (g)	Sodium (mg)	Cholesterol (mg)
Chicken Breast Boars Head Deli Meat 2oz	60	13	0	1	0	340	20
Turkey Breast Boars Head Deli Meat 2oz	60	13	0	1	0	350	35

Dairy protein
Dairy and dairy products—eleven choices:
Choose organic and no or low fat.

- Best choices are: milk, cottage cheese, and plain yogurt
- Moderate choices: cream cheese and sour cream, in moderation
- Higher in fat: butter, skim cheese, string cheese, Parmesan, Romano, and feta cheese
- Try goats or sheep milk

FOOD CHART

Dairy & Dairy Products	Calories	Protein (g)	Carbs (g)	Fat (g)	Fiber (g)	Sodium (mg)	Cholesterol (mg)
Milk							
2% (1 cup)	122	8.1	11.4	4.8	0	100	20
Fat-Free / Skim (1 cup)	91	8.7	12.3	0.6	0	130	5
Yogurt							
Plain low-fat (1/2 cup)	72	6	8	2	0	80	7
Plain whole (1/2 cup)	70	4	5.3	3.7	0	52	15
Cheese							
Cottage low-fat (1/2 cup)	100	14	6	2.5	0	440	15
Cream cheese (1 oz.)	98	2.1	0.7	9.8	0	83	31
Cream cheese reduced fat (2 Tbsp. = 1 oz.)	70	2	2	7	0	100	25
Feta (1oz.)	74	4	1.2	6	0	313	25
Mozzarella Skim (1oz.)	90	8	1	6	0	190	15
String Cheese reduced fat (1)	50	6	1	2.5	0	180	10
String Cheese regular (1)	80	7	1	6	0	210	15
Parmesan (1 Tbsp.)	50	5	0.5	3.5	0	227	9.5
Romano (1 Tbsp.)	50	4	0.5	4	0	195	10

FOOD CHART

Dairy & Dairy Products Continued...	Calories	Protein (g)	Carbs (g)	Fat (g)	Fiber (g)	Sodium (mg)	Cholesterol (mg)
Butter & Sour Cream							
Regular Butter (1 Tbsp.) Challenge brand	100	0	0	11	0	2	31
Whipped Butter (1 Tbsp.) Challenge brand	70	0	0	7	0	58	20
Sour Cream (2 Tbsp.)	62	1	1	6	0	15	13
Sour Cream (2 Tbsp.) Light Trader Joe's	40	2	2	2.5	0	20	10

Plant protein
Legumes:
Choose fresh and organic.

FOOD CHART

Legumes	Calories	Protein (g)	Carbs (g)	Fat (g)	Fiber (g)
Black Beans (1/2 cup cooked)	113.5	7.6	20.4	0.5	7.5
Chickpeas (1/2 cup cooked)	143	5.9	27.1	1.4	6
Cowpeas (1/2 cup cooked)	100	6.5	18	0.5	5.5
Green Peas (1/2 cup boiled)	67	4.3	12.5	0.2	2.4
Kidney Beans (1/2 cup cooked)	112.4	7.7	20.2	0.4	6.9
Lentils (1/2 cup cooked)	115	8.9	19.9	0.4	7.8
Lima Beans (1/2 cup cooked)	108.1	7.3	19.6	0.4	6.8
Navy Beans (1/2 cup cooked)	129	7.9	23.9	0.5	5
Pinto Beans (1/2 cup cooked)	117	7	21.8	0.4	3.4
Snap Peas (3/4 cup raw)	34	2.6	5.6	0.2	2.2
Soybeans (1/2 cup cooked)	149	14.3	8.5	7.7	3.8
Soybeans - Edamame (20)	60	5.2	4.4	2.8	1.6
Split Peas (1/2 cup cooked)	116	8.2	20.7	0.4	8.1
Winged Beans (1/2 cup cooked)	126.5	9.1	12.9	5	0

Nuts and seeds:
Choose dry and unsalted and raw when possible.

FOOD CHART

Nuts and Seeds	Calories	Protein (g)	Carbs (g)	Fat (g)	Fiber (g)
Nuts (all 1oz.)					
Almonds (dry roasted w/o salt)	170	6	5	15	3
Brazil Nuts (dried unblanched)	190	4	3	19	2
Cashews (dry roasted w/o salt)	160	4	9	13	1
Chestnuts (raw)	60	0.9	15	0.6	1.4
Coconut (raw)	99	1	4	9	3
Filberts (dry roasted w/o salt)	180	4	5	18	3
Hazelnuts (dry roasted w/o salt)	180	4	5	18	3
Hickory Nuts (dried)	184	4	5	18	2
Macadamia Nuts (dry roasted w/o salt)	200	2	4	22	2
Peanuts (dry roasted w/o salt)	170	7	6	14	2
Pecans (dry roasted w/o salt)	200	3	4	21	3
Pine Nuts (dried)	190	4	4	19	1
Pistachios (dry roasted w/o salt)	160	6	8	13	3
Walnuts	190	4	4	18	2
Seeds (all 1/4 cup)					
Flax (dry)	190	7.6	13.3	13.1	10.8
Pumpkin Seeds (raw)	228	15	5	18	2
Sesame Seeds	206	6.4	8.4	17.9	4.2
Sunflower Seeds (raw)	165	5.5	6.8	14.1	3.2

Plant protein products–seven choices:

Choose organic and made with wholesome ingredients.

- Soy butter, soy cheese, soy yogurt, soymilk, hummus, tofu, and nut butters

FOOD CHART

Plant Protein Products	Calories	Protein (g)	Carbs (g)	Fat (g)	Fiber (g)	Sodium (mg)
Soy Butter (vegan spread) Earth Balance (1 Tbsp.)	100	0	0	11	0	20
Soy Cheese (1 slice) Veggie slices – American flavor	40	3	<1	2.5	0	220
Soy Cheese (1oz.) Veggie shredded cheddar flavor	70	6	0	4	0	260
Soy Yogurt (6 oz.)	160	4	29	2	1	25
Soymilk (1 cup)	100	5	13	2	1	120
Hummus (2 Tbsp.) Wholesome Valley Organic	60	2	5	3.5	1	115
Tofu (1/5 pack = 79 g) Nasoya Organic	100	10	3	5	2	0
Nut Butters						
Peanut Butter (1 Tbsp.) Laura Scudders All Natural	105	4	3	8	1	60
Almond Butter (1 Tbsp.) Trader Joe's Creamy / Unsalted	95	4	3	9	1.5	0

Carbohydrates

Whole Grains:

Choose fresh and organic.

- Barley, oats, rice (brown, white, and wild)
- Corn and wheat (if you don't have an allergy)
- Others: amaranth, buckwheat, couscous, kamut, millet, popcorn, quinoa, rye, spelt, and triticale

Note: Serving sizes for some grains ¼ to ½ cup dry = 1 cup cooked–check the package.

FOOD CHART

Whole Grains	Calories	Protein (g)	Carbs (g)	Fat (g)	Fiber (g)
Amaranth (1/2 cup cooked)	122	4.7	21.5	2.1	4.9
Barley (1/2 cup cooked)	96.5	2	22	0.5	3
Buckwheat (1/2 cup cooked)	91	3.5	19.7	0.6	2.5
Corn (1/2 cup kernels)	90	2	18	1	3
Couscous (1/2 cup cooked)	101	3	18	0	1
Kamut (1/2 cup cooked)	110	3.5	26	1	2.3
Millet (1/2 cup cooked)	143	4.2	28.4	1.2	1.5
Oats (1/2 cup cooked)	83	3	16	2	2
Popcorn (1 cup air popped)	31	1	6.2	0.3	1.2
Quinoa (1/2 cup cooked)	127	4.5	23.4	2	2.5
Rice –white (1/2 cup cooked)	121	2	26.5	0	0.5
Rice –brown (1/2 cup cooked)	109	2.5	23	1	2
Rice – wild (1/2 cup cooked)	83	3.5	17.5	0.5	1.5
Rolled Rye (1/2 cup cooked	71	2.6	15.7	0.4	2.6
Spelt (1/2 cup cooked)	100	4	26	1	6
Triticale (1/4 cup dry)	161.2	6.3	34.6	1	0
Rolled Wheat (1/2 cup cooked)	75	3.2	12.6	1.3	1.3

Grain Products–seven choices:

Choose clean and pure grain products.

- Rice milk, rice cakes, corn thins, spelt cakes, mochi, sprouted corn tortillas, and cereals *

FOOD CHART

Grain Products	Calories	Protein (g)	Carbs (g)	Fat (g)	Fiber (g)	Sodium (mg)
Rice Milk (1 cup)	120	0.4	24.8	2	0	86
Rice Cakes (1 cake) Lundberg	70	1	16	0	1	0
Corn Thins (2 pieces) Real Foods	45	1	10	0	1	25
Spelt Puffed Cakes (1 cake) Suzie's	25	1	5	0	1	0
Sprouted Corn Tortilla (2) Food 4 Life Flourless	120	3	23	2	3	10
Mochi (1 2X2 piece) Grainassance	120	2	25	1	3	35

* Cereals – see nutrition facts in the Diva Reduction Safe Cereal List
– PART SIX

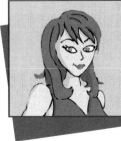

"Bread is not all bad and can even be a good part of your daily diet, unless you eat the whole loaf. You can find other grain products that are good for you too–like tortillas, pasta, and cereal. See our Paw guide on the next page. ...."

"......This, as well as the Paw Guide for Choosing Safe Cereals (found in this section), and the Paw Grain Products Guide (found in PART FOUR) will give you what you need to make informed choices with all grain products."

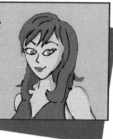

Paw "10 Directives to Bread" Guide

1. They should be made with whole grain like amaranth, barley, millet, oats, quinoa, rice, rye, spelt, and wheat.
2. They can contain added legumes, nuts, and seeds–if they are pure.
3. They are best if they are organic and sprouted or stoned ground.
4. Flour-made breads are okay, as long as it is not white flour.
5. Gluten-free, wheat-free, and yeast-free are good options.
6. They can have multiple ingredients but should be made with only clean and pure ingredients
7. They should be high in protein, fiber, and other nutrients, and low in fat.
8. They should be low in preservatives and additive-free.
9. They should have limited or no sugar, sodium, or oils, however, if they do contain these they should come from natural and healthy sources.
10. The following is a list of recommended breads. They are calorically dense (a slice or two equals anywhere from 100 to 250 calories and 2-20 grams of fiber) and they require refrigeration.

Paw "10 Directives to Bread" Guide

The Good Bread List
- Food For Life Ezekiel Bread (flourless)
- Food For Life Raisin Pecan (wheat and gluten-free)
- Food For Life China Rice Bread (wheat and gluten-free)
- Health Seed Organic 100% Rye Bread with Flax, Pumpkin and Sunflower Seeds (wheat-free)
- Health Seed Organic Spelt, with Organic Flax, Pumpkin and Sunflower Seeds (yeast-free)
- Pacific Bakery Yeast-Free Spelt–Cinnamon Raisin Organic Bread
- Julian Bakery (wheat-free)
- Bible Recipe Bread–Complete Protein Bread (organic and sweet-free, yeast and wheat-free)
- Manna Bread–Complete Protein Bread (all sprouted, wheat, yeast and sweet-free)

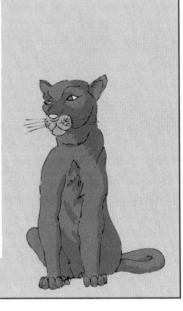

Vegetables:
Choose organic–raw and fresh is best.

FOOD CHART

Fresh Vegetables	Calories	Protein (g)	Carbs (g)	Fat (g)	Fiber (g)
Artichoke (1 boiled)	60	4	13.5	0.2	1.5
Asparagus (1/2 cup, boiled)	23	2.3	4	0.3	1.5
Beets (1/2 cup slices, boiled)	37	1.4	8.5	0	1.7
Broccoli (1/2 cup chopped, boiled)	22	2.3	4	0.3	2
Brussels Sprouts (1/2 cup, boiled)	30	2	6.8	0.4	3.4
Cabbage (1/2 cup shredded, boiled)	16	0.7	3.6	0.2	1.8
Carrot (1 medium, raw)	31	0.7	7.3	0.1	2.3
Cauliflower (3 florets, raw)	13	1.1	2.8	0.1	1.3
Cauliflower (1/2 cup, cooked)	14	1.1	2.5	0.3	1.7
Celery (1/2 cup diced, raw) approx 1-2 stalks	10	0.5	2.2	0.1	1
Corn on-the-cob (1 ear, boiled)	83	2.6	19.3	1	2.9
Cucumber (1/2, raw)	20	0.8	4.4	0.2	1.5
Eggplant (1/2 cup, cubed, boiled)	13	0.4	3.2	0.1	1.2
Green Beans (1/4 cup, raw)	25	1	5	0	3
Jicama (1 cup slices, raw)	46	1	11	0	6
Butterhead Lettuce (1 cup, shredded)	5	0.5	1	0.1	0.4
Iceberg Lettuce (1 cup, shredded)	18	1.4	2.8	0.3	1.4
Loose Leaf Lettuce (1 cup, shredded)	10	0.7	2	0.2	1
Romaine Lettuce (1 cup, shredded)	9	0.9	1.3	0.1	1

FOOD CHART

Fresh Vegetables continued...	Calories	Protein (g)	Carbs (g)	Fat (g)	Fiber (g)
Mushrooms (1 medium)	4	0.6	0.6	0.1	0.2
Onion (1/2 cup, chopped)	36	0.8	8.6	0.1	1.2
Parsley (1/2 cup, chopped, raw)	10	0.7	2.1	0.1	1.3
Chili Peppers (1 Tbsp., raw)	4	0.2	0.9	0	0.1
Green/Red Bell Peppers (1/2 cup, chopped, raw)	14	0.5	3.2	0.1	0.8
Potato (8 oz., baked)	220	4.7	51	0.2	2.2
Canned Pumpkin (1/2 cup)	41	1.3	9.9	0.3	3.4
Radishes (1/2 cup, sliced, raw)	10	0.4	2	0.3	1.3
Scallions (1/2 cup, chopped, raw)	16	0.9	3.7	0.1	1.2
Shallots (1 Tbsp.)	7	0.3	1.7	0	0.2
Spinach (1/2 cup, boiled)	21	2.7	3.4	0.2	2
Acorn Squash (1/2 cup, cubed, baked)	57	1.1	14.9	0.1	2.9
Butternut Squash (1/2 cup, cubed, baked)	41	0.9	10.7	0.1	2.9
Hubbard Squash (1/2 cup, cubed, backed)	51	3	11	0.6	2.9
Spaghetti Squash (1 cup, boiled, or baked)	45	1	10	0.4	2.2
Zucchini (1/2 cup slices, boiled)	14	0.6	3.5	0.1	1.3
Sweet Potato (4 oz., baked- approximately 1/2)	117	2	27.7	0.1	3 . 7
Tomato (1 raw = 1/2 cup)	26	1.1	5	0.4	1.6
Yams (1/2 cup, boiled, or baked)	79	1	18.7	0.1	2.7

Fruits:
Choose organic–raw and fresh is best.

FOOD CHART

Fresh Fruit	Calories	Protein (g)	Carbs (g)	Fat (g)	Fiber (g)
Apple 1 (5 oz. with skin)	81	0.3	21.1	0.5	3
Apricots 3 (4 oz.)	51	1.5	11.8	0.4	2
Avocado 1/2 (3 oz.)	162	2	7.5	15.4	2.1
Banana (1 med, without skin)	105	1.2	26	0.5	3
Blackberries (1 cup)	75	1	18.4	0.6	7.2
Blueberries (1 cup)	81	1	20.5	0.6	3.3
Cantaloupe (1 cup, cubed)	56	1.4	13.4	0.5	1.3
Cherries Sweet (1 cup, without pits)	104	1.7	24	1.4	1.6
Cranberries (1/2 cup)	23	0.2	6	0.1	2
Grapefruit 1/2 (4 oz.)	37	0.7	9.5	0.1	0.7
Grapes (1 cup, American)	58	0.3	15.8	0.3	0.6
Guava 1 (3 oz.)	46	0.7	10.7	0.5	4.9
Honeydew (1 cup, cubed)	60	0.8	15.6	0.2	1.4
Kiwifruit 1 (2½ oz.)	46	0.8	11.3	0.3	2.6
Lemon 1/2 (1 oz., without skin)	8	0.3	2.7	0.1	0.6
Lime 1/2 (1 oz., without skin)	10	0.2	3.5	0.1	0.7
Mango 1/2 (3 ½ oz.)	67	0.5	17.6	0.3	2.1
Nectarine 1 (5 oz.)	67	1.3	16	0.6	2.2
Orange 1 (4 ½ oz.)	62	1.2	15.4	0.2	3.1
Olives 1 (large)	5	0	0.3	0.5	0.1
Papaya 1/2 (5½ oz.)	59	0.9	14.9	0.2	2.6
Peach 1	37	0.6	9.7	0.1	1.4
Pear 1 (6 oz.)	98	0.7	25.1	0.7	4.3
Pineapple (1 cup, cubed)	76	0.6	19.2	0.7	1.9

FOOD CHART

Fresh Fruit cont...	Calories	Protein (g)	Carbs (g)	Fat (g)	Fiber (g)
Plum 2 (4½ oz.)	73	1	17.2	0.8	2
Pomegranate 1/2 (3 oz.)	52	0.7	13.2	0.2	2.8
Raspberries 1 cup	60	1.1	14.2	0.7	8
Strawberries 1 cup	45	0.9	10.5	0.6	3.9
Tangerine 1 (3 oz.)	37	0.5	9.4	0.2	1
Watermelon (1 cup, cubed)	51	1	11.5	0.7	0.6

Dried fruits—four choices

- Figs, raisins, dates, and prunes

  You can have more dried fruit if they are pure (check the ingredients).

FOOD CHART

Dried Fruit	Calories	Protein (g)	Carbs (g)	Fat (g)	Fiber (g)
Figs 3 (2 oz.)	143	1.7	36.7	0.7	5.2
Figs 3 (organic, white)	110	1	26	0	5
Prunes 5 (1½ oz.)	100	1.1	26.3	0.2	3
Raisins (1/2 cup)	218	2.3	57.4	0.3	3.9
Dates 5 (1½ oz.)	114	0.8	30.5	0.2	3.5

Herbs, spices, and other plant foods:

Herbs and spices are great for adding flavor but have many other benefits as well. See Herbs and Spices in PART SEVEN.

FOOD CHART

Herbs, spices, and other plant foods	Calories	Protein (g)	Carbs (g)	Fat (g)	Fiber (g)
Basil (2 tsp., ground)	7.5	0.5	1.9	0.1	1.2
Black Peppercorns (2 tsp., ground)	10.9	0.5	2.8	0.1	1.1
Garlic (1 oz. / 3 cloves, raw)	42.1	1.8	9.4	0.1	0.6
Cinnamon (2 tsp., ground)	11.9	0.2	3.6	0.2	2.5
Cayenne and Red Chili Peppers (2 tsp.)	11.2	0.4	2	0.6	1
Cilantro (2 Tbsp., fresh)	0.5	0	0.1	0	0.1
Dill (2 tsp., dried)	5.1	0.4	1.1	0.1	0.3
Ginger (1 oz., fresh)	19.6	0.5	4.3	0.2	0.6
Mustard Seeds (2 tsp., seeds)	35	1.9	2.6	2.2	1
Parsley (2 Tbsp., fresh)	2.7	0.2	0.5	0.1	0.3
Rosemary (2 tsp., dried)	7.3	0.1	1.4	0.3	0.9
Turmeric (2 tsp., ground)	16	0.4	3	0.4	1

Extra Sweeteners—four choices
- Agave nectar, applesauce (organic, sugar-free), fruit spreads (natural), and honey—all in moderation

FOOD CHART

Extra Sweeteners	Calories	Protein (g)	Carbs (g)	Fat (g)	Fiber (g)	Sodium (mg)
Agave nectar (1 Tbsp.)	20	0	11	0	2.8	0
Applesauce - sugar free (1/2 cup)	60	0	13	0	2	20
Fruit Spread (1 Tbsp.)	36	0	9	0	0	0
Honey (1 Tbsp.)	70	0	17	0	0	0

Fats and Oils

Good sources of quality fat include unrefined vegetable sources or oily fish
- Oils like olive, safflower, sesame, soybean, and sunflower
- Others include: flax oil, canola oil, extra virgin olive oil, soy oil, wheat germ oil, walnut oil, and hemp seed oil
- Oily fish: salmon, mackerel, sardines, and tuna

Notes on Fats:
- Traces of fats can be found in fresh fruits and vegetables.
- Higher amounts of good fats are in many foods like avocados, olives, nuts and seeds.
- Most protein-rich foods like eggs, beef, dark poultry meat, fish, dairy, and dairy products contain fat. Some contain good fats and cholesterol and some contain essential fatty acids.
- Fats are in most salad dressings, spreads, sauces, and dips.
- Look carefully to find man-made food products that contain good fats.

FOOD CHART

Oils	Calories	Protein (g)	Carbs (g)	Fat (g)	Sat. Fat (g)	Mono. Fat (g)	Poly. Fat (g)	Cholesgterol (mg)
Olive Oil	120	0	0	13.6	1.8	10	1.2	0
Safflower Oil	120	0	0	13.6	1.2	1.7	10.1	0
Sesame Oil	120	0	0	13.6	1.9	5.4	5.7	0
Soybean Oil	120	0	0	13.6	2	3.2	7.9	0
Sunflower Oil	120	0	0	13.6	1.4	2.7	8.9	0
Cooking Spray (1 second spray)	7	0	0	0	0	0	0	0

FOOD CHART

Salad Dressing Regular (all 2 Tbsp.)	Calories	Protein (g)	Carbs (g)	Fat (g)	Sodium (mg)
Balsamic Vinaigrette (Trader Joe's)	100	0	5	11	270
Blue Cheese	154	2	2	16	335
Caesar Dressing (Gerard's)	140	1	1	15	360
Caesar- Romano Dressing (Trader Joe's)	180	0	0	20	150
French	134	0	5	13	427
French Vinaigrette	177	0	1	20	184
Italian	137	0	3	14	231
Oil & Vinegar (Newman's)	150	0	1	16	150
Red-Wine & Olive Oil (Litehouse)	130	0	4	12	135
Thousand Island	118	0	5	11	218

FOOD CHART

Salad Dressing Low Fat (all 2 Tbsp.)	Calories	Protein (g)	Carbs (g)	Fat (g)	Sodium (mg)
Balsamic Vinegar	20	0	4	0	0
Blue Cheese	50	1	6	2	310
French Tomato	60	0	8	3	280
Italian	32	0	2	3	236
Russian (low calorie)	46	0	9	1.5	283
Thousand Island (low calorie)	49	0	5	3.3	306

FOOD CHART

Mayonnaise (all 1 Tbsp.)	Calories	Protein (g)	Carbs (g)	Fat (g)	Sodium (mg)
Mayonnaise (regular)	90	0	0	10	90
Mayonnaise (reduced fat)	20	0	2	2	125
Mayonnaise (vegan light)	35	0	0	3.5	65
Soy Mayo	35	<1	1	3.5	115

FOOD CHART

Other	Calories	Protein (g)	Carbs (g)	Fat (g)	Sodium (mg)
Salsa Muir Glen Organic (2 Tbsp.)	10	0	2	0	130
Marinara Melissa's Organic (1/2 cup)	80	2	8	4.5	380

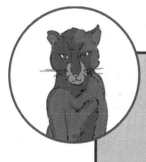

Some packaged foods are okay to use occassionally, but should be examined thoroughly.
Canned and frozen foods like:

- Canned tuna, legumes, olives, and soups
- Frozen fruits and vegetables with a few ingredients
- Salad dressing, sauces, seasonings, and dips

Diva Reduction Safe Cereal List

Here is a list of cereals (hot and cold) MY DIVA DIET endorses.
They:
- Are all gluten-free.
- Have no trans fats, saturated fat, or cholesterol.
- Are very low in or have no preservatives or additives.
- Contain less than 2 grams of sugar.
- Are very low in or have no sodium at all.
- Are made from the whole grain–most are not from processed grains.
- Are not made from white or wheat flour.
- Are not made from any flour at all.

Hot
1. Arrowhead Mills Organic Steel Cut Oats - Organic, Wheat-Free, Vegetarian
   ¼ cup = 160 calories; 6 g protein; 27 g carbs; 3 g fat;
   8 g fiber; 0 mg sodium; 0 g sugar
2. Old Fashioned Quaker Oats - 100% Natural
   ½ cup dry = 150 calories; 5 g protein; 27 g carbs; 3 g fat;
   4 g fiber; 0 mg sodium; 1 g sugar
3. Ancient Harvest Quinoa - Wheat Free, Gluten Free, Organic
   ¼ cup dry = 166 calories; 5 g protein; 30 g carbs; 3 g fat;
   3 g fiber; 5 mg sodium; 1 g sugar
4. Ancient Harvest Quinoa Flakes - Organic, Gluten Free Kosher
   .33 cup = 134 calories; 4 g protein; 23 g carbs; 0 g fat;
   2.6 g fiber; 4 mg sodium; 1 g sugar
5. Lundberg Cream of Rice Cereal - Gluten Free, Organic, Vegan
   ¼ cup dry = ½ cup cooked = 150 calories; 3 g protein; 32 g carbs; 1.5 g fat;
   3 g fiber; 0 mg sodium; 0 g sugar
6. Pocono Cream of Buckwheat - Wheat & Gluten Free, Organic
   .25 cup = 140 calories; 2 g protein; 36 g carbs; 0 g fat;
   1 g fiber; 0 mg sodium; 0 g sugar

Cold

7. Nu-World Foods Amaranth Berry Delicious Gluten Free, Milk-Free, Corn-Free, Egg-Free, Nut-Free, Soy-Free, Kosher, Organic

    1 cup = 86 calories; 4 g protein; 18 g carbs; 1 g fat;

    3 g fiber; 3 mg sodium; 1 g sugar

8. Erewhon Organic Crispy Brown Rice – Gluten-Free, Organic, Kosher

    1 cup = 110 calories; 2 g protein; 25 g carbs; 0.5 g fat;

    0 g fiber; 160 mg sodium; 2 g sugar

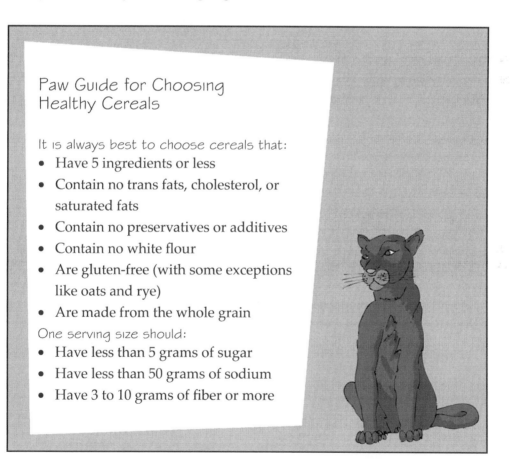

Paw Guide for Choosing
Healthy Cereals

It is always best to choose cereals that:
- Have 5 ingredients or less
- Contain no trans fats, cholesterol, or saturated fats
- Contain no preservatives or additives
- Contain no white flour
- Are gluten-free (with some exceptions like oats and rye)
- Are made from the whole grain

One serving size should:
- Have less than 5 grams of sugar
- Have less than 50 grams of sodium
- Have 3 to 10 grams of fiber or more

Reading Labels

"The Food and Drug Administration (FDA) is responsible for assuring that foods sold in the United States are safe, wholesome, and properly labeled. This applies to foods produced domestically, as wells as foods from foreign countries."

"The Nutrition Labeling and Education Act (NLEA), which amended the Food, Drug & Cosmetic (FD&C) Act requires most foods to bear nutrition labeling and requires food labels that bear nutrient claims and certain health messages to comply with specific requirements. (Regulations are frequently changed)."*

Food Labels include the following:
Dietary Guidelines for Americans
This is found on the nutrition panel. It was designed by the United States Department of Agriculture (USDA) in 1980 and is updated every five years.

Nutrient Descriptors and Claims
This is found on the front of the package and is designed to get your attention–to encourage you to buy the product. Commonly used words are, "light", "low fat", "no trans fats", and many more.

Health Claims
Health claims are common practice when foods that are packaged and/or man-made food products are marketed. Food companies use health problems (often caused by poor diet), certain nutrient deficiencies, the importance of certain nutrients, and the dangers of certain additives and preservatives to convince you to buy their products.

---

* Food Label Resources:
- FDA U.S. Food and Drug Administration
- Center for Food Safety and Applied Nutrition
- CFSAN/Office of Nutrition, Labeling, and Dietary Supplements, April 2008
  http://www.cfsan.fda.gov/guidance.html

Health Claims Include:

- Calcium and osteoporosis

  Claim: Adequate calcium reduces the risk of osteoporosis.

- Fat and Cancer

  Claim: Low-fat foods may help lower the risk for developing some types of cancer.

- Saturated fat and cholesterol and coronary heart disease

  Claim: Foods low in saturated fats and cholesterol may reduce risk of heart disease.

- Fiber (containing vegetables, fruits, and grains)

  Claim: Fiber reduces the risk of heart disease and certain cancers.

- Omega 3–Fatty Acids

  Claim: Omega-3 reduces the risk of coronary heart disease.

- Sodium and high blood pressure

  Claim: A low-sodium diet reduces blood pressure.

- Folate and birth defects

  Claim: Adequate folate intake may reduce a woman's risk of having a child with a neural tube defect.

Note: Products that make health claims are subject to certain regulations set by the FDA. However, we really don't know how strict they are and the degree of enforcement is unlcear.

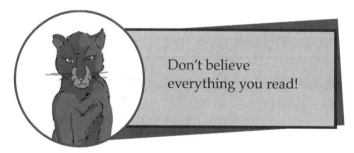

Don't believe
everything you read!

Organic Labeling

On food labels, products using the term "organic" must meet the following guidelines:

- "100% Organic" means it must contain only organically produced ingredients.
- "Organic" means it must contain at least 95% organically produced ingredients.
- Processed products that contain at least 70% organic ingredients can use the phrase "Made With Organic Ingredients".

The Nutrition Facts

The nutritional panel is on the back of most packaged and man-made food products. This includes both mandatory and voluntary information.

List of Ingredients

Ingredients for all foods (including standardized foods) must be listed on the food label. The label must also list the FDA-certified color additives by name. Ingredients are listed by weight, in descending order.

Food Allergies

Since January 2006, food manufacturers must also disclose whether products contain any of the top eight food allergens (milk, eggs, fish, shellfish, peanuts, tree nuts, wheat, and soy). However, the label does not specifically address gluten. "Gluten Free" labeling is currently voluntary, but many food companies add it to their labels. This is due to the new trend of gluten-free foods becoming more popular.

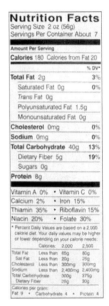

"To really know what you are getting when you buy a packaged and/or man-made food products–DO YOUR HOMEWORK–your health depends on it."

FDA Label Definitions

Here are some terms used in food labeling:

- "Calorie free" means less than 5 calories per serving.
- "Cholesterol free" means less than 2 mg of cholesterol per serving.
- "Enriched" or "fortified" means a food has been nutritionally altered, usually to add certain nutrients to the product.

- "Fat free" means 0.5 g of fat per serving.
- "Fresh" indicates foods used in their raw state.
- "High" indicates that a serving of the food contains 20% or more of the daily value for a particular nutrient.
- "Lean" means 10 g of fat, 4 g saturated fat, and 95 mg of cholesterol per serving.
- "Less" signifies that a food contains 25% or less of a nutrient than a comparable food.
- "Low" means little or few. Whether it is calories, certain nutrients, or minerals, each company has its own standard for what is considered low.
- "More" indicates that a serving of food contains at least 10% more of the daily value of a nutrient than a comparable food.
- "Salt free" or "sodium free" means less than 5 mg per serving.
- "Sugar free" means less than 0.5 g of sugar per serving.

Key words and phrases to look for when reading labels:
- Additives: a substance added directly to food during processing, for preservation, coloring, or stabilization
- Artificial: made by human skill, as opposed to natural
- Genetically modified: adjusted, shaped, reformed; tempered or altered the quality of something
- Kosher: allowed by law or regarded as correct or proper (used to describe food that has been prepared so that it is fit and suitable under Jewish law)
- Natural: relating to nature, present in or produced by nature, rather than being artificial or created by humans
- Organic: relating to or employing agricultural practices that avoid the use of synthetic chemicals in favor of naturally occurring pesticides, fertilizers, and other growing aids
- Pasteurization: to expose food (as milk, cheese, yogurt, beer or wine) to an elevated temperature for a period of sufficient time to destroy certain microorganisms, as those that can produce disease or cause spoilage or undesired fermentation of food, without radically altering taste or quality
- Preservatives: chemical substances used to preserve foods from decomposition
- Processed: converted into a marketable form by a special process
- Refined: free from impurities (i.e. refined sugar)

Food Additives

Here is a short list and information on some commonly used food additives in food products today. There are too many to address them all.

#1. Aspartame:
Aspartame is an artificial sweetener (the white powder in the little blue packets) commonly used in "diet foods" like soft drinks, drink mixes, gelatin desserts, low calorie frozen desserts, etc. Aspartame (Equal, NutraSweet), is a chemical combination of two amino acids and methanol, and has recently been linked to cancer and neurological problems.

#2. Baking Powder, Baking Soda:
Baking powder and baking soda are both leavening agents used in cooking baked goods. These items produce carbon dioxide, which causes a baked good to "rise". Baking soda is pure sodium bicarbonate, which means it needs an acidic ingredient like yogurt, buttermilk, chocolate, or honey to produce carbon dioxide. Baking powder contains sodium bicarbonate and has an acidic ingredient already included in it.

MR. BAKERMAN

#3. Citric Acid:
Citric Acid is found in citrus fruits and vegetables, and is a weak organic acid. It is also a natural preservative, antioxidant, and is used to add an acidic or sour taste to foods and soft drinks. This acid can be used as a thickening and stabilizing agent, and is found in ice cream, jelly, chocolate milk, and infant formula. Citric acid is most concentrated in lemons and limes. Citric acid is safe, cheap, versatile, and widely used.

#4. Corn Syrup:
Corn syrup is used as a sweetener and as a thickener. It can be found in many food items like candy, toppings, syrups, snack foods, and imitation dairy foods. Corn syrup is a thick liquid consisting mostly of dextrose and treated with cornstarch containing acids or enzymes. Corn syrup is high in calories, promotes tooth decay, is used in foods with little nutritional value, and by itself has no nutritional value.

#5. Dextrin:
Dextrin is a food additive that acts as a rising agent or binder, a stabilizer, and a thickener. Dextrin can be found in foods like dairy products, processed cheeses, blends of butter and margarine, cereals, pre-cooked pastas, soybean products, and batters. Dextrin is produced by acidic hydrolysis of potato starch.

#6. Fructose and High Fructose Corn Syrup:
Fructose is one of three simple blood sugars that are primarily found in honey, fruits, and some vegetables. While fructose is a very important source of energy for many body processes, over-consumption can overwhelm the body's ability to process it, causing the excess to be converted to fats in the bloodstream (triglycerides). The presence of excess triglycerides has been linked to an increased risk of heart disease, appetite de-regulation (feelings of dissatisfaction or hunger which may lead to weight gain), and potential insulin resistance (which leads to the onset of type II diabetes).

High fructose corn syrup (HFCS) is pure corn syrup (100% glucose–another simple sugar) added to glucose, which has undergone a process that increases the amount of fructose in the final product. There are different grades of HFCS, each primarily for a different purpose.
- HFCS 90: 90% fructose, 10% glucose (used in baked goods),
- HFCS 55: 55% fructose, 45% glucose (used in soft drinks), and
- HFCS 42: 42% fructose, 58% glucose (used in sports drinks).

#7. Hydrogenated and Partially Hydrogenated Oil:
Hydrogenation is the process of heating oil and passing hydrogen bubbles through it. By hydrogenating oil, either partially or fully, you are creating a solid and dense consistency. Because of this consistency, and because it is cheap, hydrogenated and partially hydrogenated oil is a favorite butter substitute among food producers. The American obesity epidemic began when oils like coconut oils were replaced by partially hydrogenated oils.

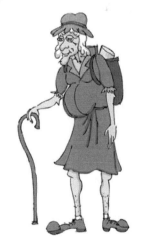

TRANNY GRANNY

#8. Lactic Acid:
Lactic acid is found in sour milk products like koumiss, leban, yogurt, kefir, and some cottage cheeses. It is found in Spanish olives, frozen desserts, and carbonated beverages. Lactic acid is also found in various processed foods. It is used as a preservative, controls acidity, and is used as a fermentation booster in rye and sourdough breads. This is a safe acid that occurs in almost all living organisms.

#9. MSG (monosodium glutamate):
MSG is a flavor enhancer used in soups, salad dressings, chips, frozen entrees, and restaurant foods. MSG brings out the flavor in many foods, but this so-called "treat for our taste buds" allows companies and restaurants to reduce the amount of real food ingredients. Studies have shown that MSG fed to mice destroyed nerve cells in their brains. Some nutrition experts claim that people are sensitive to MSG and reactions include: headaches, nausea, weakness, burning sensations in the back of the neck and arms, wheezing, changes in heart rate, and difficulty breathing.

#10. Saccharin:
Saccharin is an artificial sweetener found in "diet" products, soft drinks, sugar packets, and fountain drinks at restaurants. In animal studies saccharin has caused cancer of the bladder, uterus, ovaries, skin, blood vessels and other organs. In 1977 the FDA wanted to ban saccharin because of these animal studies, but congress intervened and permitted its use as long as there was a warning label. In 2000 saccharin was removed from the list of cancer causing chemicals and Congress passed a law removing the warning label. As a result, use of saccharin in soft drinks and other foods will likely increase, and so will the incidence of cancer.

#11. Sodium Chloride:
Sodium chloride, also known as salt, is a flavoring used in most processed foods, cured meats, soups, snack chips, crackers, and others. Salt acts as a preservative, adds flavor, masks bitter flavor, and fosters expected textures, but the levels of sodium in our diets today are probably one of the most harmful substance in our food supply. Diets high in salt increase blood pressure, which increases the risk of heart attack and stroke. Many companies are reducing the sodium content in their food products because of the growing concerns regarding salt and how it affects health.

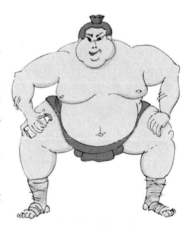

SODI SUMO

262

#12. Sodium Nitrite, Sodium Nitrate:
Sodium nitrite is a preservative, a coloring, and a flavoring in bacon, ham, frankfurters, lunchmeats, smoked fish, and corned beef. This is what keeps the red color in meats–otherwise meats like hot dogs and bacon would look gray. Sodium Nitrate is used in dry cured meats because it breaks down into nitrite. Potent cancer-causing chemicals can form with the addition of nitrite into food.

#13. Soybean and Cottonseed Oil:
Soybean and cottonseed oils are, most of the time, hydrogenated or partially hydrogenated, which makes them very unhealthy. Cottonseed oil is now used in manufacturing potato chips and other snack foods, despite being originally intended for candle production. Cottonseed oil might contain high amounts of pesticide residues, but sufficient testing has not been done. Soybean oil, sometimes hydrogenated or partially hydrogenated, is sold and exported around the world and used in a wide variety of processed foods. Soybean oil has also been effective as an insect repellent.

#14. Starch, Modified Food Starch:
Starch and modified food starch are thickening agents used in soups, gravies, and baby foods. Starch is the fundamental component of flour, potatoes, and corn, and is used to thicken many foods. Chemists created modified food starch because starch by itself does not dissolve in cold water. Modified food starches sometime replace fresh and nutritious ingredients.

#15. Sugar:
Sugar primarily comes from sugar cane and sugar beets and goes through a refining process. Table sugar (granulated white sugar), which is stripped of all vitamins, minerals, fiber, amino acids and trace elements during the refining process, is pure sucrose.

Sugar can affect health in a myriad of ways–suppress the immune system, cause free radical formation in the bloodstream, produce a significant rise in triglycerides and increase in total cholesterol, cause hypoglycemia, kidney damage, produce an acidic stomach, overstress the pancreas, increase risk of Crohn's disease and ulcerative colitis, increase the amount of fat in the liver, cause hormonal imbalance, increase in the body's fluid retention, lead to many mineral deficiencies, speed up aging, cause headaches, including migraines, promotes tooth decay and periodontal disease. Sugar also contributes

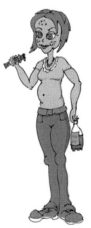

SHOOG

263

to hyperactivity, anxiety and depression, diabetes, osteoporosis, weight gain and obesity. And this is the abbreviated list.

#16. Yeast:
There are over a hundred varieties of yeast in nature, known as "wild yeast", to make breads and other baked foods. There is also yeast known as "brewer's yeast", and this is used for making beer, wine, ale, and bread. Yeast has the outstanding ability to convert sugar to carbon dioxide and alcohol. Yeast has been used since at least as far back as the year 2000 B.C.

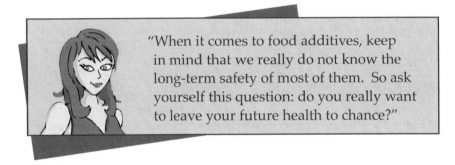

"When it comes to food additives, keep in mind that we really do not know the long-term safety of most of them. So ask yourself this question: do you really want to leave your future health to chance?"

Diva Food Test & Paw Label Guide

Here is a quick six-question test you can perform when deciding what to eat. This is where the quality and purity of calories are determined. When choosing a food and/or food product, you must be able to answer "yes" to three or more of the six questions listed below. Using this food test will ensure that your food choices fit into the MY DIVA DIET program for fat loss and better health.

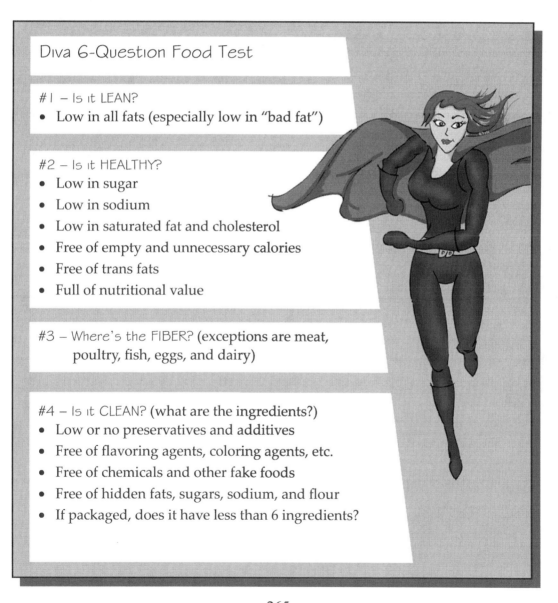

Diva 6-Question Food Test

#1 – Is it LEAN?
- Low in all fats (especially low in "bad fat")

#2 – Is it HEALTHY?
- Low in sugar
- Low in sodium
- Low in saturated fat and cholesterol
- Free of empty and unnecessary calories
- Free of trans fats
- Full of nutritional value

#3 – Where's the FIBER? (exceptions are meat, poultry, fish, eggs, and dairy)

#4 – Is it CLEAN? (what are the ingredients?)
- Low or no preservatives and additives
- Free of flavoring agents, coloring agents, etc.
- Free of chemicals and other fake foods
- Free of hidden fats, sugars, sodium, and flour
- If packaged, does it have less than 6 ingredients?

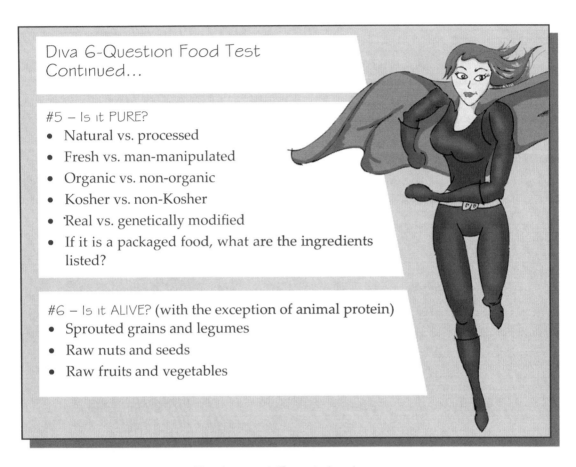

Diva 6-Question Food Test
Continued...

#5 – Is it PURE?
- Natural vs. processed
- Fresh vs. man-manipulated
- Organic vs. non-organic
- Kosher vs. non-Kosher
- 'Real vs. genetically modified
- If it is a packaged food, what are the ingredients listed?

#6 – Is it ALIVE? (with the exception of animal protein)
- Sprouted grains and legumes
- Raw nuts and seeds
- Raw fruits and vegetables

Packaged Food Analysis

There are seven main questions you should ask when you are considering packaged foods that are manipulated or man-made.

1. Who made it?
2. How was it made?
3. How many ingredients are in it?
4. What is in it (what are the ingredients)?

You should also wonder:

5. Where was the product made?
6. What kind of factories and equipment were used?
7. What are the conditions and practices of the company that made, processed or packaged the product?

When you examine labels of man-made food products or any packaged food here are some other things to know and do:

- Read the nutrition facts and know that it only gives part of the picture.
- Know that some products have zero nutrition.
- Read the list of ingredients and know that:
  - The order of the ingredient tells you a lot about a particular product.
  - The ingredients are listed in descending order–from most to least.
  - It does not tell you exactly how much of each ingredient is used.
- Choosing packaged foods and man-made food products is NOT always "black and white".
  - There will always be Best – Moderate – Marginal – Worst.
- Use the Paw Ingredients Label Guide to help you deal with the number of ingredients and determine how many are appropriate.
- If you can't pronounce the ingredient, you probably shouldn't purchase that product.
- Don't buy into the health claims–pure and wholesome foods offer the best health benefits and are safe!

Paw Ingredients Label Guide

Number of Ingredients	Signals
1	Ideal
3	Excellent
5	Probably OK
6-9	May need further analysis
10-19	Could be a problem
20-29	Caution
30 +	Stay away!

MY DIVA DIET Restaurant Eating Guide: 52 Tips
Diva Reduction and Diva Maintenance

Restaurant Dining Meal Problems
- Too much fat, sodium, and sugar
- Too much white flour
- Too much alcohol
- Too many unfamiliar foods
- Too many people handling your food
- Overeating and late-night eating

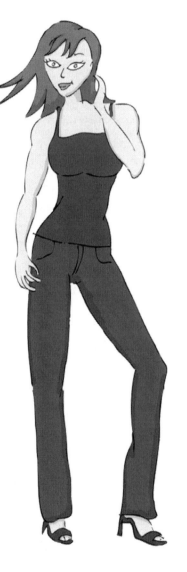

Remember—you are the customer, so don't be afraid to ask questions and make requests. Before ordering, always ask how a dish is prepared and what ingredients it contains. Then think of how you can substitute or eliminate something in your order.

Beverages
#1 Water is best to drink. Try adding a slice of lemon or lime if you need flavor.

- Stay away from sodas and other sugary types of drinks, including juices, unless they are freshly squeezed.
- Coffee and tea are fine - no cream or sugar!

#2 Limit alcohol.

- Choose wine over exotic drinks like margaritas, piña coladas, and mai tais.
- Beer is not recommended.

Appetizers
#3 Choose your appetizers wisely, if at all.

- Appetizers are usually high in fat and calories and often contain "forbidden" foods.
- Don't forget that you have a meal coming—maybe you don't really need that appetizer.

#4　At some restaurants you can order a good appetizer that can actually be your main course. That way you won't overeat and it will save you money. Just tell the server to bring it out when the other entrées come.

#5　Go light on all types of dips. Salsa is good but watch the chips and guacamole.

First Course

#6　Stay away from the bread. It is not only a poor choice but it will make you too full to eat the healthier part of your meal, like protein and veggies. Some bread every so often is okay, but eat it sparingly.

#7　Stay with broth-type instead of cream-type soups (a good choice would be vegetable soup or tomato soup).
- Cream soups are full of fat, sodium, white flour, and other unknown ingredients.
- Broth soups can be high in sodium but they have fewer calories, and it's easier to figure out their ingredients.

#8　Salads and salad dishes are great, just order dressing on the side so you can control the amount you use.

#9　Be adventurous when choosing a salad: try a beet salad instead of a house or mixed-green salad. You will get more variety in raw vegetables and thus more nutrients.

#10　Be careful of crumbled cheese toppings added to salads.
- Blue cheese, feta, goat, fontina, and other cheeses may taste good but they are very high in calories and fat grams.
- Ask for crumbled cheese on the side so you can control the amount.

#11　Always choose low or non-fat dressings for all salads and veggies.
- Vinegar and lemon are good non-fat choices.
- Balsamic vinegar and olive oil are high in nutrients—just control the amount of oil.

Main Course

#12 Fish is an excellent entrée.
- Choose halibut, salmon, trout, tuna, whitefish, red snapper, and sea bass.
- Avoid swordfish, shark, and catfish.
- Avoid shellfish like crab, lobster, and shrimp.
- Avoid clams, mussels, oysters, and scallops.

#13 Poultry is always a safe and lean choice.
- Try to choose white meat over dark meat.
- Remove the skin (it's full of fat). It's easy to take off.

#14 Beef is all right—just choose lean cuts, and trim off the visible fat. Try to restrict beef to once or twice a month.
- Good choices are filet, New York, top sirloin, porterhouse, and T-bone.
- Lamb and veal are also fine, occasionally.

#15 Limit duck and avoid pork. Pigs are cute but they do not have the same digestive system as cows. And they not only eat the food they are given, but also anything else they can find.

#16 Watch out for foods that are not just plain fish, poultry, or beef (i.e. chicken chow mein, lobster ravioli, seafood pasta, etc.). These kinds of dishes have many ingredients like oil, butter, cream, white flour, and salt and are very high in calories. You can't really calculate what you are eating and it is safe to say that you are getting more ingredients than the protein you need. Better to choose your main course as a single item.

#17 Bean dishes are great, just watch what is used in preparing them like lard, oil, and too much cheese.

#18 Corn tortillas are better than flour. Make sure they are not fried.

#19 Potatoes are great only if they are plain and either baked or boiled. Watch the toppings—butter, sour cream, chives, and bacon. Order your potato plain with the toppings on the side, be selective with topping choices, and use your toppings sparingly.

#20 Rice is good, but most restaurants cook rice with added oil and salt. The exceptions are Chinese and Japanese restaurants, where you can order plain rice. Skip the rice at other restaurants unless you know what is in it and how it was prepared. Find a health conscious restaurant that serves plain brown rice.

#21 Pasta and pasta dishes are okay occasionally. It is better to choose ones with marinara instead of cream sauce (like fettuccini Alfredo) due to the high fat content. A good idea is to use pasta as a side dish rather than a main dish (unless it is a special "cheat" night).

#22 All fresh vegetables are great.
  • Watch for veggies that are prepared with oil, butter, sauce, and salt.
  • Eat vegetables *al dente*, which ensures the highest nutritional value.

#23 Make sure the food you order is fresh—not processed, canned, or frozen. Eat organic foods if possible. And try to seek out restaurants that serve kosher!

#24 Stay away from all fried foods.

#25 Stay away from all breaded foods.

#26 Make sure the food you order is baked, broiled, grilled, poached, or steamed.
  • Stir-fry is acceptable.
  • Stay clear of microwave cooking if at all possible.

#27 Have the chef go light on oil when preparing all foods. If oil is being used, ask if it is olive oil or an oil low in saturated fats and with no trans fats. Find out—it is your body and your money.

#28 Do not salt your food. There is plenty of sodium in your food when you are dining out, even when you are careful with ordering.

#29 All spices, herbs, and vegetables are great for enhancing the flavor of foods. Look for garlic, onions, leeks, basil, pepper, oregano, sage, and cinnamon, just to name a few. Hopefully, you have chosen a restaurant with a chef who is an expert at seasoning his dishes the healthy way.

#30 Go light on all sauces or gravies (or avoid them completely).
- Sauces are full of fat, sodium, white flour, and other ingredients you don't need.
- If you do use them, ask for sauces and gravies on the side so you can control the amounts.

#31 Go light on condiments like mayonnaise and ketchup.
- Mustard and horseradish are good choices.
- Teriyaki, barbecue, and tomato sauce are okay on occasion.
- If you must use soy sauce, use the light kind.

#32 Go light on all oils and nuts, or any dish with these products.

#33 Go light on butter, cheese, sour cream, and other dairy products. A little Parmesan, Romano, and feta cheese goes a long way in flavor!

Desserts
#34 Cheesecake, fruit cobblers, pies, crème brûlée, and other desserts taste yummy but are very high in calories and are mainly white flour, sugar, and fat.
- Try fruit desserts like mixed berries, which are full of fiber and antioxidants. If you need the extra sweets, add a little whipped cream or vanilla ice cream on the side.
- Sorbet is another option, even with the sugar content. There are a variety of flavors and they taste great!
- A little spumoni or green tea ice cream is okay.

Note on desserts:
It is dessert, after all, so go for it—just don't go for it every time. If you need to splurge and fruit or sorbet is not sufficient, then try ordering one big dessert and sharing it with your party or date.

Breakfast
#35 Ask that your eggs and omelets be made with whites only, with minimal butter or oil. That way, you cut the fat in half.
- Omelets are great if you add a variety of vegetables.
- For extra flavor, try adding some salsa and other herbs to your eggs.
- Egg Beaters are okay.

#36 Try to stay away from pancakes, waffles, crepes, etc. They are mainly white flour and sugar!

#37 Try to avoid bacon, ham, and sausages. These foods are high in fat, sodium, and cholesterol, and include many additives and preservatives—and you never know the quality of a restaurant product. Turkey sausage is okay occasionally.

#38 Skip bread and baked goods like donuts, pastries, and muffins—you'll regret eating them later.
- A piece of rye or sourdough toast or a bagel is fine once in a while.
- You can add a small amount of natural fruit spread if you need that sweet flavor.

#39 Avoid hash browns, breakfast potatoes, and French fries. Potatoes are a great food but these are all fried in oil, so they are very high in fat even if they are cooked with a good fat. Some restaurants use frozen potatoes. If you are going to eat these it should only be once in a while, and you should find out if the potatoes are fresh or frozen, as wells as what kind of oil is used to cook them in.

#40 Go light on sugar, molasses, syrup, jams, and jellies. A little honey, agave nectar, or real-fruit "fruit spread" are better options.

Lunch

#41 Sandwiches and wraps are more healthful if they are ordered on whole-wheat or multigrain breads, pita bread, flat bread, or tortilla wraps (like rice or corn tortillas) with low-fat meats, poultry, and fish.
- Be aware that deli meats are not fresh meats—they are processed, with many preservatives and additives. If you do select a deli sandwich occasionally, choose only lean chicken and turkey deli meats low in sugar, sodium and gluten-free.
- Add flavor and nutrients with veggies like lettuce, tomatoes, green peppers, and olives.
- Ask your sandwich-maker to skip calorie pitfalls like cheese and avocado.
- Go light on the mayo—mustard is much better.

#2   Salad for lunch is a good idea and a great way to get your vegetables and protein.
  • You can usually find a tasty chicken Caesar salad—just watch the dressing and skip the croutons (white flour).
  • Chinese chicken salad is good too—just watch the amount of dressing and skip the chow mein noodles (white flour).
  • A mixed-green or beet salad with a side of chicken breast is a great idea.
  • A good tuna salad also makes for a nice healthy lunch.

#43 Soup for lunch is great if you can find one that is full of fresh vegetables. A good chicken soup with lots of vegetables would work well here—just watch for ingredients like noodles (which are made with white flour and too much sodium).

#44 It's okay to have a hamburger for lunch once in a while. Try to find burgers made with lean beef or ground turkey (kosher is best), or a vegetarian type. To boost nutritional value, skip the bread and add a side salad.

Other Tips and Notes

#45 To avoid overindulgence or overeating at a restaurant, try eating an apple an hour before dining out. This will help cut your appetite and control your food choices.

#46 If you know you will be dining out for dinner, plan on eating below your calorie goal from your other meals that day. Avoid skipping meals, which may make you overeat at the restaurant.

#47 If you are trying to avoid alcohol but would still like to feel included with others who are drinking, ask that your water or beverage also be served in a wine glass.

#48 Restaurants tend to serve large portions. Try splitting a meal with a dining partner to control portion size.

#49 Order from the a la carte menu. Separate food items will not come with extra sides like rice, potatoes, fries, or beans. This will help with portion control.

#50 If you are eating at a buffet (which is not a good idea), use a salad plate. Smaller portions equal fewer calories (and fewer poor food choices).

#51 Eat your food at a nice slow pace.
   • When you eat slowly, your body will tell you when you are full and need to stop.
   • Use chopsticks often, as this will force you to eat more slowly.
   • Try to stop eating a few bites before you feel full.

#52 Finally, remember that you are dining out—splurging once in a while is good for you, so relax and enjoy yourself.

Bon appétit!

Paw Mini Menu Restaurant Guide

American:
- Turkey, beef, or veggie burger (no bread)
- With side salad (lowfat dressing) or with side of veggies (no sauce, no oil)

Barbecue:
- Chicken or beef (grilled)
- With baked potato (plain)
- With side salad (lowfat dressing)

Chinese:
- Lettuce wraps or string bean chicken (skip the sauce)
- With side of steamed white rice

Indian:
- Tandori chicken with veggies
- With side of steamed rice

Italian:
- Grilled fish or beef (sauce on side)
- With sides of pasta and veggies

Japanese:
- Teriyaki chicken/salmon (a la carte)
- With veggie roll or cucumber salad
- With side of steamed white rice

Mexican:
- Chicken fajitas or chicken taco (all the veggies, no cheese)
- With side of black beans (no cheese)

Steakhouse:
- Small filet mignon (sauce on side)
- With baked potato (plain) and side of veggies or side salad (lowfat dressing)

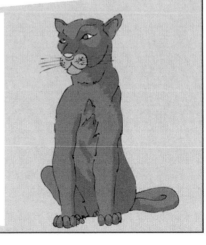

*Keep in mind most restaurants do not use organic or kosher products. Een when you order specific items, you will probably only get part of what you want. For example; your chicken order (unless it states chicken breast) is usually white and dark meat mixed. They also always use large amounts of salt, oils, and sauces in the preparation.

Fast Food

The topic of fast food is always a consideration in any diet program. Fast food places are all over, however, some are much better than others, even if they offer no-fat and "so-called" healthier menu items.

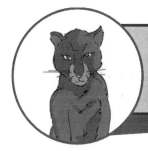

Do yourself and your family a big favor. Do your own research on fast food items and be extremely selective when you decide which drive-through to visit and which item to order.

Twelve Problems with fast food:

Ask these questions:

1. Where does the meat come from? And is it really meat?
2. How was the animal (meat) raised, slaughtered, and processed?
3. What is really in the food? Is it real?
4. Is it fresh? Or is it frozen, canned, dehydrated, or freeze-dried?
5. How many additives and preservatives like sugar, fat, salt, and white flour (and their derivatives) do they use?
6. How many chemicals are used?
7. How many flavor enhancers are in the food. And what do they use to enhance flavor and appeal?
8. How many fake and cooked fats like hydrogenated oils are used.
9. Is there any nutritional value?
10. Where is the fiber?
11. How many calories are you about to eat?
12. What are the conditions and practices of the fast food chain?

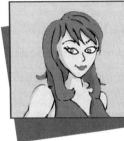

"If you are not up-to-date on the damage fast food can do to your figure and your health; the threat it poses to our children; and the horrific things it does to animals, our food, the environment; and the danger it places on the people that work in the fast food industry..."

...... try watching Eric Schlosser's "Fast Food Nation" (read the book too) and Morgan Spurlock's "Super Size Me."

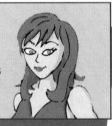

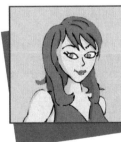

"Poor quality meat (meat derived from animal cruelty and unsafe methods of processing) and other standard food items are just found not in fast food places—they are also in many of the restaurants at which we frequently dine at."

Paw Fast Food Five Guide

5 Tips:

1. Avoid fast food.
2. Use fast food only as an "I haven't eaten all day" solution.
3. Choose the healthiest menu items.
4. Don't super-size – eat small portions or share.
5. Your best bet: Go to your local health food store and choose lean dishes from the deli or find a place to get a healthy protein shake or smoothie (these are fast meals but much healthier)!

5 Places:

1. Baja Fresh
2. Panda Express
3. Quizno's
4. Subway
5. Taco Bell

*Check websites for nutrition facts

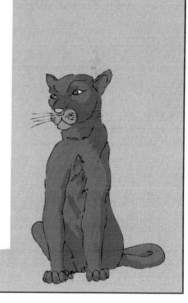

Note on fast food:

If you must eat fast food, we are providing you with five places to eat and a few meal options. They are not perfect meal choices but are close to the MY DIVA DIET criteria. Don't make them a "habit".

Baja Fresh

www.bajafresh.com

Items: Chicken Original Taco, Steak Original Taco, Mahi Mahi Taco grilled, Baja Ensalada with Charbroiled Chicken (try light or small portion of dressing), or side of black beans (go light on the added cheese)

Notes: Items are between 200-360 calories; 2-10 grams of fat; 2-26 grams of fiber.

TIPS: Baja Fresh has ingredients that are much better than most fast food chains, however, their burritos could feed three people. The Baja Chicken Burrito has 790 calories, 38 grams of fat, and 2140 milligrams of sodium. So sharing would be a good idea here. The complimentary chips are 210 calories and have 9 grams of fat. Watch the guacamole because it has 34 grams of fat. The Chicken Tortilla Soup is extremely high in sodium (2760 mg) as are many of their other items.

Panda Express Chinese

www.pandaexpress.com

Items: Steamed Rice, Mixed Veggies, String Bean Chicken Breast, Black Pepper Chicken, or Mushroom Chicken

Notes: Items are between 90-390 calories; 2-12 grams of fat; 2-4 grams of fiber.

TIPS: Panda Express usually uses a lot of sauces on their food items, which means higher fat and sodium—skip the ones with sauce and choose plain steamed veggies and rice. They also use the dark meat of the poultry in many of their dishes. Stay clear of Potstickers and Egg Rolls where you will waste 200 calories on white flour, 8-12 grams of fat, and 300 to 400 milligrams of sodium for one small serving.

Quizno's

www.quiznos.com

Items: Veggie Sub (small—without cheese and dressing), Honey Bourbon Chicken Sandwich (small with dressing), Chicken Caesar Chopped Flat Bread Salad, Roast Chicken with Honey Mustard Flat Bread Salad

Notes: Items are between 250-310 calories; 4-15 grams fat; 4-6 grams of fiber. Dressings from Quizno's (per package) are on average 300-500 calories; 30-50 grams of fat; 500 to 1200 milligrams of sodium; 2-20 grams of sugar—try the Balsamic vinaigrette instead.

Subway

www.subway.com

Items: 6" Oven Roasted Chicken Breast Sandwich,   6" Veggie Delight Sandwich, Chicken or Turkey Breast Wrap, Grilled Chicken & Baby Spinach Salad, or Fit Mini Sub - Turkey Breast

Notes: Items are between 140-310 calories; 3-7 grams of fat; 3-10 grams of fiber.

TIPS: Quizno's and Subway: The great thing about Quizno's and Subway is that they are health conscious companies that cater to healthy people by providing them with fresh ingredients. Choose low-fat dressing, but if you decide to have regular dressing don't use it all. Eliminate bread or only eat half of it. Be careful with the cheese, avocado, mayo, and oil commonly used on a wrap or sandwich.

Taco Bell
www.tacobell.com
Items: Bean Burrito, Burrito Supreme–Chicken, Crunchy Taco (Fresco Style), or Ranchero Chicken soft taco (Fresco Style)
Notes: Items are between 150-330 calories; 4-10 grams of fat; 3-8 grams of fiber.
TIPS: At Taco Bell, ask for the "Fresco Style"; they will replace the cheese and sauce with salsa (diced tomatoes, with onions and cilantro). It will significantly reduce the calories, fat grams, and sodium and will eliminate trans fats!

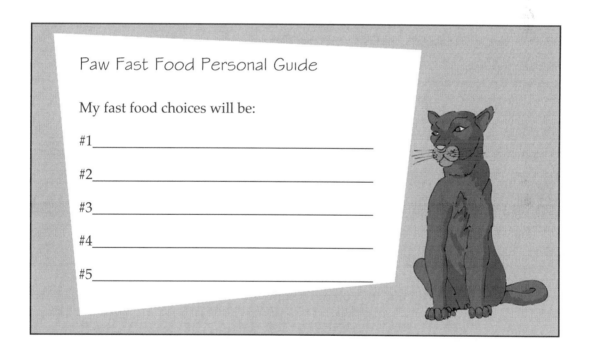

Paw Fast Food Personal Guide

My fast food choices will be:

#1_____

#2_____

#3_____

#4_____

#5_____

Interesting fact to chew on:
According to the research done by Eric Schlosser of "Fast Food Nation". "In 2001, Americans spent more than $110 billion on fast food. Americans now spend more money on fast food than on higher education, personal computers, computer software, or new cars."

Twenty Shocking Facts About Fast Food
Did you know?

1. One Burger King Whopper has 628 calories! That's just about half of your daily calories.

2. One Carl's Jr. Western Bacon Cheeseburger has 1570 milligrams of sodium. That's almost all the sodium you need in a day.

3. The Breakfast Jack, served at Jack in the Box, has 220 grams of cholesterol.

4. There are 1,010 calories and 2580 milligrams of sodium in the 6 Piece Garlic Parmesan Twists served at Round Table Pizza.

5. The Bacon Ultimate Cheeseburger from Jack in the Box has 77 grams of fat!

6. One medium chocolate shake from Dairy Queen has 133 grams of carbohydrates. That's almost all the carbohydrates you need in a day—and they are bad carbohydrates!

7. At Wendy's, the Big Bacon Classic Burger has 260 calories coming from fat!

8. The Chicken Pot Pie from KFC has 40 grams of fat, and 770 calories!

9. The McDonald's Deluxe Breakfast has a shocking 1190 calories!

10. A Strawberry Slush at Sonic has 185 grams of sugar!

11. A Double Quarter Pounder with Cheese at McDonald's has 20 grams of saturated fat!

12. At Carl's Jr., the Catch Fish sandwich has 3927 milligrams of sodium!

13. The Pancakes with bacon served at Whataburger has 118 grams of carbohydrates.

14. The Double Whopper with cheese at Burger King has 185 milligrams of cholesterol.

15. Hardee's 2/3 lb. Bacon Cheese Thickburger has 96 grams of fat!

16. The Double Chili Burger at Carl's Jr. has 962 calories!

17. There are 20 grams of sugar in the Western Bacon Six Dollar Burger served at Carl's Jr.

18. The Super Sonic No. 1 at Sonic has 596 calories from fat.

19. At Wendy's, the Chicken BLT Salad with toppings has 19 grams of fat.

20. A basket of 21 Crunchy Shrimp pieces at Long John Silver's has 105 milligrams of cholesterol.

PART SEVEN

Valuable Information

You gain strength, courage, and confidence by
every experience in which you really
stop to look fear in the face.
~ Eleanor Roosevelt

Calories: Friends or Foes?

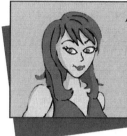

"One of our goals here at MY DIVA DIET is to free you from any hang-ups concerning food. Another goal is to clear up some common misconceptions about dieting. Dieting should be neither difficult nor confusing; instead, it should be a positive aspect of life with which we strive to be at peace."

In this section we'll tackle the following topics:
The Definition and Function of Calories
Understanding Basal Metabolic Rate (BMR)

Like the word *diet*, the word *calorie* gets a bad rap. As women, it seems we are afraid and constantly worried about calories and their power over us.

Let's take a little journey so we can better understand what calories are and how they work in the human body. If we learn the facts, we'll be on our way to understanding the truth about calories.

FACT #1
What is a calorie?
According to Webster's dictionary, a calorie is "a unit for measuring heat". The scientific way of defining it is this: "a calorie is the amount of energy, or heat, it takes to raise the temperature of one kilogram of water by one degree Celsius". Basically, calories are just energy.

FACT #2
What do calories do?
Human beings (and animals) need energy to survive and they require energy from food. Our food has three main components: protein, carbohydrates, and fats. They are digested in the intestine, then broken down into their basic units: proteins into amino acids, carbohydrates into sugars, and fats into fatty acids. The body uses these basic units to build substances it needs for growth, maintenance, and activity.

FACT #3
What is BMR?

BMR stands for Basal Metabolic Rate. BMR is basically the amount of energy your body needs to maintain normal body function. This includes the function of vital organs like the heart, lungs, brain and nervous system, liver, kidneys, sex organs, muscle, and skin, and accounts for about 60-70% of calories burned in a day. The amount of energy required by these processes must be met before any of those calories can be used for food digestion and physical activity.

FACT#4
What can affect one's BMR?

One's BMR can be influenced by a combination of genetic and environmental factors: genetics, age, gender, weight, body surface area, body fat percentage, body temperature and health, external temperature, glands, diet, and exercise.
Here a few explanations.

Genetics:
Some people are born with faster BMR, some with slower.

Age:
BMR reduces with age. Because of the increase in cellular activity (cells undergoing division), BMR is highest during the growth spurts that take place during childhood, adolescence, and pregnancy. BMR peaks at age twenty for males and females, then decreases by about 2% per decade throughout life. This decline during adulthood may result partly from a decrease in physical activity and the subsequent loss of muscle tissue.

Gender:
Due to a greater percentage of muscle mass (lean tissue) and a lower body fat percentage, men generally have a higher BMR than women.

Body fat percentage:
The lower the body fat percentage, the higher the BMR. Since the male body has a lower body fat percentage–they generally have a 10-15% higher BMR than women.

Female vs. Male BMR and Muscle Mass:
Muscle tissue is, metabolically, highly active even at rest, whereas fat tissue is not. Thus, lean body mass (LBM) greatly influences a body's energy requirements and, in conjunction, its nutrient needs. An increase in muscle mass, for both males and females, will elevate BMR.

So, while gender is an influential factor, the fact that we are women is not necessarily the culprit when it comes to our lower BMR. Instead, a woman's lower BMR is due to a smaller proportion of muscle mass to fat. This direct relationship is a main reason that strength training is so important in a weight-loss program. Regular strength training can have a positive effect on the development and protection of lean body mass.

Starvation – Restrictive Dieting:
Metabolic rate can drop to as low as 20-30% during a period of starvation and restrictive low-calorie dieting. This drop is due to the body's effort to conserve energy (and its eventual loss of lean tissue) by slowing its BMR. This slowing process is a natural protective mechanism that conserves fat stores when a food shortage occurs. Because of this, consumption of fewer calories than required to sustain BMR will be counterproductive, and can actually cause body fat levels to increase.

Exercise:
Exercise can increase BMR and, depending on intensity and duration, the metabolic rate may remain elevated for several hours afterward. During sustained, large-muscle exercises like running and swimming, people can generate metabolic rates that are ten times higher than their resting values. Exercise will also increase your muscle mass, which will then increase your BMR.

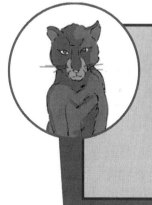

This is why many top athletes can consume high amounts of calories and still maintain low body fat. The value of exercise cannot be overlooked–it is Factor #5 in the MY DIVA DIET program! Exercise is critical for both short and long-term fat loss; it prevents obesity, poor posture, muscle and bone loss, pre-mature aging, depression, and many other health issues, and it facilitates ultimate fitness levels; physically, mentally, and emotionally.

Keeping this information in mind, the next step is to calculate calories according to personal BMR and activity level. As women, our BMR is naturally lower than that of men, so we shouldn't eat as much as they can (or do). Although gender equality is an important issue, food consumption is one aspect of life in which we shouldn't try to compete with men–we should not eat more than we need. And, if we swing in the other direction and don't eat enough, our predicament is just as grim.

While we can't change our genetics, age, gender, height, or (in most cases) our environment, we *can* change our body composition. We can decrease our body fat and increase our lean body mass (LBM). Changing our body composition is done through proper diet and exercise–two things that will directly impact BMR. By changing our body composition, we can increase our BMR. You will learn more about Body Composition in PART EIGHT. Certain things to consider when it comes to the potential for women to increase LBM:

- Due to the hormonal make-up of women, we can only gain a certain amount of muscle mass.
- Excessive muscle mass may result in a less feminine appearance, so it is important to decide how much is appropriate for you.

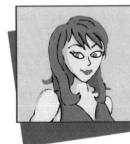

"Since women are limited in how much lean body mass we can and in some cases want to have, the total amount of calories we can consume in a day should always be limited–unless we join the Marines, start running marathons, or find ourselves qualifying for the Olympics!"

If you are a little confused at this point just remember one thing: calories are your friend, and a friend is:
- Someone who is not your enemy
- Someone you can trust
- Someone you can count on
- Someone who sticks by your side no matter what
- Someone who defends or supports you
- Someone who would never hurt you intentionally

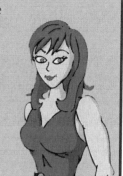

Not all calories are created equal. We get our calories from three main sources, each with a different function and energy potential.

Paw Nutrient Functions Basic Guide

Protein: The Cellular Building Block
- Is a main component of bones, muscles, organs, glands, cartilage, skin, and blood
  - Blood has three functions: transportation, regulation, and protection
- Aids in development, maintenance, and repair of all body tissue
- Aids in formation of hormones, enzymes, and other body chemicals
- Is important for growth and development during childhood, adolescence, and pregnancy

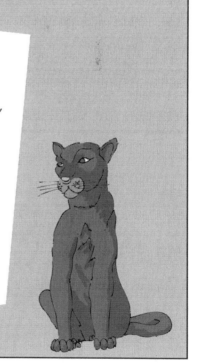

Paw Nutrient Functions Basic Guide
Continued....

Carbohydrates: Chief Energy Source
- Provide energy for all bodily functions and muscular exertion
- Are the only source of energy for the brain, nervous system, and red blood cells
- Help regulate protein and fat metabolism
- Are required to break down fats in the liver
- Help regulate blood glucose levels
- Assist in digestion and assimilation of other nutrients
- Provide nutrients for bacteria in the intestinal tract that aid digestion

Fats: Supply Necessary Nutrients
- Provide essential fatty acids from mono- and poly-unsaturated fats
- Aid in growth, maintenance of healthy skin, vitamin absorption, and regulation of bodily functions
- Provide energy (as the most concentrated fuel source)
- Aid in heart and brain health, prevention of certain cancers, and reduction of other ailments like depression, inflammation, and blood pressure

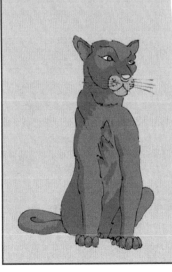

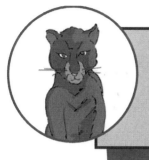

Although calories are necessary to sustain life and each nutrient has a particular function for health & fitness, an excess of any of these will be converted by the liver and stored as fat. Even good calories, when consumed in large amounts, can end up doing harm.

FACT #6:

Energy Balance:

The caloric energy of a particular food depends on how much protein, carbohydrate, and fat it contains. Most foods contain mixtures of these three nutrients and are classified by which is most predominant. A food rich in protein, like beef, actually contains a lot of fat, while a carbohydrate-rich food like grain contains small traces of both fat and protein.

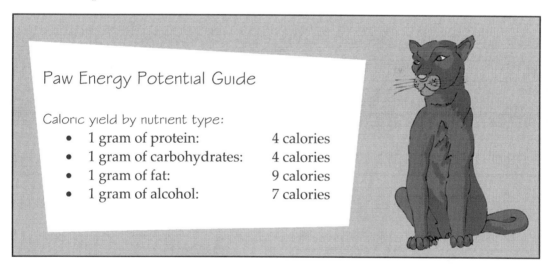

Paw Energy Potential Guide

Caloric yield by nutrient type:

- 1 gram of protein: 4 calories
- 1 gram of carbohydrates: 4 calories
- 1 gram of fat: 9 calories
- 1 gram of alcohol: 7 calories

Like many well-designed machines, the body stores energy for future use. Its primary means of storage is fat, or adipose tissue, which lies beneath the skin and surrounds the organs. You can think of fat and its caloric potential as a gas tank for the body. But, unlike a gas tank, the body's capacity to accumulate an energy reserve is almost limitless. Calories consumed in excess of the body's needs are stored as fat (in your fat cells–around your internal organs and visible places like your hips, butt, thighs, etc.).

FACT #5:

Weight control is a question of energy balance:

Energy in = Energy expended = WEIGHT STABLE
Energy in > Energy expended = WEIGHT GAIN
Energy in < Energy expended = WEIGHT LOSS

It sounds simple, but in reality it is somewhat complex. Calculating the correct amount of calories (energy) to consume each day, then trying to figure out the proper nutrient ratio for a healthy & fit body can be like trying to do your first science project. That's why we've done the math for you at MY DIVA DIET! This section will teach you about calories and their overall importance in health & fitness so you can embrace them as your friend.

Why Restrictive and Unbalanced Diets Don't Work

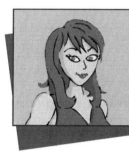

"There is no quick-fix for fat loss, optimal health, and longevity. If there were, we would have figured it out by now! But, the good news is that there is a way, and we can help you down that path."

MY DIVA DIET is not interested in attacking any particular product or program by name. However, we do want to expose the truth about the $50 billion "health & fitness" industry. Many of the programs marketed today are basically gimmicks full of false promises, magic potions, and misleading propaganda. Most of these counter-productive systems result in yo-yo dieting and can be quite dangerous.

"No sensible diet will ever compromise your physical or mental health for the sake of looking good."

Our hope is that the next time another quick-fix diet system surfaces, you will know better than to believe the hype, or at least that you'll think twice before you waste your time, money, and health.

Commonly used formulas for fat-loss diets:
Liquid Diets
- Most are low-calorie diets
- Less than 1000 daily calories translates to starvation
- Do you plan on living only on liquids for the rest of your life?

Low-Calorie Diets

- Any diet of less than 1000 daily calories will slow your metabolism and put you at a nutritional risk that could lead to health problems
- Reduced energy levels
- Decrease in water weight, not necessarily fat

High-protein, Low-carbohydrate, High-fat Diets

- Too much protein can put undue stress on your kidneys and other internal organs which could lead to health problems
- High amounts of calories from protein, if not used for their intended purpose, can convert to body fat
- Fat burns in the flame of a carbohydrate–thus you need carbs to help metabolize fat
- Carbohydrates are needed for energy and exercise
- Carbohydrates are necessary for brain function–without them you will inhibit your ability to concentrate, calculate, and coordinate, and your memory and moods will be affected
- High-protein, low-carbohydrate diets can put you into a state of ketosis, which is not healthy and can lead to loss of lean body mass
- Carbohydrates provide fiber, whereas fats and animal protein contain no fiber
- Low-carbohydrate diets often result in water loss, not fat loss
- High-fat intake converts easily to body fat and is unhealthy

Low-Protein, High-Carbohydrate, No-Fat Diets

- Protein is necessary for every cell in the body so a lack of protein can cause deficiencies and health problems
- Protein is needed for muscle growth, maintenance, and repair
- Excess carbohydrates can convert to body fat
- High carbohydrates can cause bloat and puffiness
- It is impossible to avoid dietary fats–fat is found in many foods naturally
- Some fat is necessary for health and vitality–too little fat can cause a deficiency in fat-soluble vitamins and essential fatty acids

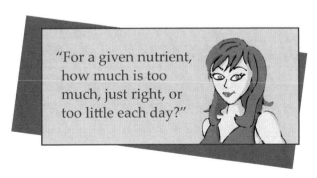

"For a given nutrient, how much is too much, just right, or too little each day?"

This question is where the real debate begins amongst fitness professionals and diet gurus. MY DIVA DIET has designed a simple chart of highs and lows for the average female. This chart is not intended for those with special circumstances, athletes, growing children, or pregnant or menopausal women.

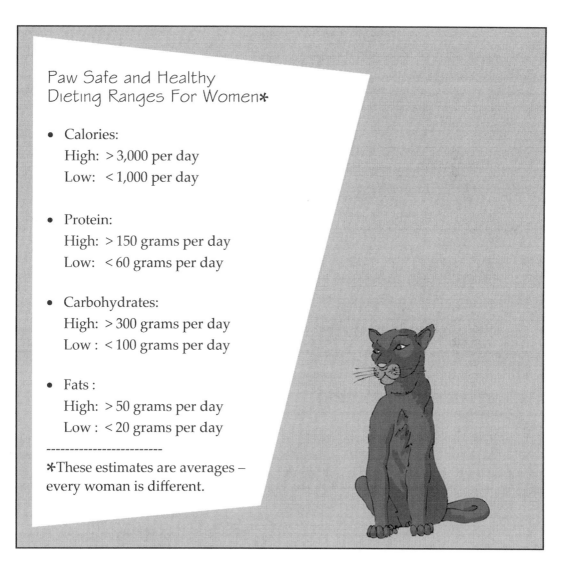

Paw Safe and Healthy
Dieting Ranges For Women*

- Calories:
  High: > 3,000 per day
  Low: < 1,000 per day

- Protein:
  High: > 150 grams per day
  Low: < 60 grams per day

- Carbohydrates:
  High: > 300 grams per day
  Low : < 100 grams per day

- Fats :
  High: > 50 grams per day
  Low : < 20 grams per day

----

*These estimates are averages –
every woman is different.

Other Diet Programs

One Meal per Day Diet

- Eating smaller meals throughout the day is important for utilizing calories more efficiently and creating a constant energy level; both are important in the overall fat-loss and better health equation

- Eating one meal (or two) per day does not generate a steady blood glucose level

- Eating one meal per day promotes over-eating especially if that one meal is eaten at night—starving all day causes you to eat everything in sight

- Eating one meal per day promotes bad food choices because excessive hunger will cause you to be less selective with your food choices

One Type of Food Diet

- Too much of one type of food causes nutritional imbalances and deficiencies which can lead to health issues both short- and long-term

- All-fruit diets result in water-weight loss, not fat loss

- This type of diet can eventually lead to muscle loss, which is directly linked to your metabolism. Since more lean-body mass means a more active metabolic rate, you will lose fat more quickly by maintaining and/or increasing your LBM.

Processed, Packaged, and Man-Made Food Diet

- Nutritional value is reduced or eliminated when foods are altered from their natural state

- When you cut calories, you lose weight. However, if you only eat packaged, processed, and man-made foods, your weight-loss potential will be limited by food quality, and your health may be compromised

- Our bodies cannot properly metabolize most additives and preservatives

- Our goal is to lose fat, gain health, function and feel better, and live longer. Consuming unnatural foods is detrimental to this goal.

One Part of the Equation Diet

- Diet programs that tell you to JUST eat less, or eat better, or eat low glycemic foods, or eat only raw foods, or eat six meals per day, or just cut the sugar, or just exercise, etc. may be good ideas and very helpful to your goals of fat loss and better health— but they don't give you the complete dieting picture.

- Providing only part of the diet equation is like presenting a puzzle with some of the pieces missing–will you ever complete the entire picture? NO!

#1 – Poor Health

Since most quick-fix diets restrict calories or do not allocate the proper nutrient ratio (protein, carbohydrates, and fat), and even completely eliminate important vitamins, minerals, and fiber, they put you at a nutritional risk. This sets the stage for a number of health problems during your diet, in the immediate future, and further down the line.

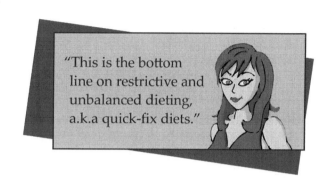

"This is the bottom line on restrictive and unbalanced dieting, a.k.a quick-fix diets."

#2 – Dehydration

Some quick-fix diets promote low-carbohydrate intake. However, most of the weight lost in this manner consists only of glycogen and water. Since the human body is over 60% water, this kind of diet may lead to dehydration. Dehydration can cause fatigue, crankiness, stiff joints, headaches, nausea, aches, electrolyte imbalances, and much more. Severe dehydration can cause seizures, coma, or even death.

The other problem with water-weight loss is that women are deceived into believing that they're losing fat. In reality, once carbohydrate intake resumes (even the good carbs) and the water weight is restored, women mistakenly believe they've regained all the "fat" they had lost on their diet programs.

#3 – LBM Reduction

Reduction in muscle mass is a common result of any type of low-calorie, low-carbohydrate, or starvation program. In fact, as muscle mass is lost, metabolism slows. A daily intake of less than 1000 calories is considered starvation, and the human body will automatically try to salvage body fat just for survival.

#4 – Decrease in Energy

When calories are restricted, especially carbohydrates, the body's main source of energy is limited. This energy is needed for the body and the brain to function properly. Otherwise, you'll begin to feel tired, cranky, and mentally slow. You also will not have the energy you need to be active and exercise. Calories do so much for your body–they provide energy, life, vitality, and so much more–why would you give that up?

#5 – Body Fat Increases

- Any type of restrictive or unbalanced diet is a recipe for failure. The hype behind quick-fix diets is often unsubstantiated–they are based on gimmicks and full of false promises.

- Since most quick-fix diet programs offer ways to lose weight fast with no regard for health and safety, the results will always be questionable.

- After trying a quick-fix diet program, any attempt to resume normal, proper eating patterns often causes us to regain more weight than we lost.

- Regaining weight creates desperation, which often causes us to seek another quick-fix. This process eventually leads to chronic yo-yo dieting, which is a. vicious, unhealthy, frustrating, expensive, and dangerous cycle.

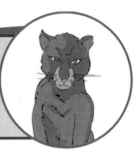

Don't trust Dr. Pill, and don't follow the example set by Nurse Gimmick–fat loss, optimal health, and longevity require proper diet and exercise; followed by a lifestyle change.

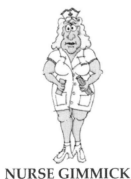

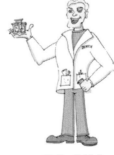

NURSE GIMMICK   **DR. PILL**

Herbs & Spices

Herbs and spices are a great addition to any diet program. They enhance flavor, improve the appeal, and increase the nutritional value of any dish. They also replace the need for other ingredients like fat, sugar, sodium, and flour.

These are some benefits of herbs and spices:
- Low in calories and fat
- Provide a variety of vitamins and minerals
- Provide fiber, antioxidants, phytonutrients, antimicrobial properties, and anti-inflammatory potential

The properties found in herbs and spices promote the following:
- Natural defense against infections
- Joint health
- Heart health
- Balanced blood sugar
- Digestive health
- Weight control
- Enhanced memory
- Enhanced detoxification

  For example:
  - Liver supporters: milk thistle and dandelion
  - Blood cleansers: red clove and burdock
  - Metabolism boosters: cumin, coriander, dill, mustard seed, and cinnamon

"Herbs & spices are often a forgotten treasure, and here at MY DIVA DIET we think you should know more about them."

Wars have been fought and countries discovered because of "treasured" spices. Marco Polo's accounts of his trip to China in the late 1200s told of the spice trade in unknown lands, and many Europeans went in search of the exotic indulgence. In the fifteenth through the seventeenth centuries, Spanish, English, Portuguese, and Dutch traders competed in the Far East for dominance in the spice trade, and by the late 1800s America became involved. America's first millionaires made their money in spices.

Herbs: These are leaves of low-growing shrubs. Popular herbs include parsley, chives, marjoram, thyme, basil, caraway, dill, oregano, rosemary, savory, sage, and celery leaves.

Spices: These come from the bark (cinnamon), root (ginger, onion, garlic), buds (cloves, saffron), seeds (yellow mustard, poppy, sesame), berries (black pepper), or fruit (allspice, paprika) of tropical plants and trees.

Frequently Used Herbs & Spices:

Basil:
The word basil is derived from the old Greek word *basilikohn*, which means "royal". Basil has many medicinal purposes including aiding in digestion and helping with nausea and motion sickness. Dried basil is also good for the respiratory system and can be used to treat nose and throat infections. Fresh basil contains folic acid, and dried basil is a good source of potassium, iron, and calcium.
TIP: Try adding basil to different foods like meats, poultry, pasta, pizza, salad, and soups.

Black Pepper:
The pepper plant is a smooth woody vine that can grow up to thirty-three feet in hot and humid climates. After three to four years of growth, peppercorn berries are produced, and this is the part of the plant that gives us pepper. Freshly ground black pepper improves digestion, promotes sweating and urination, and helps stimulate the breakdown of fat cells.
TIP: Try adding fresh-ground pepper to foods like beef, poultry, salad, and soup.

Cayenne Pepper:
For more than seven thousand years, cayenne pepper has been prized for its healing qualities. Cayenne is helpful for the entire digestive system as well as the heart and circulatory system. It is high in vitamins A, B, C, and K, and very high in organic calcium, potassium, manganese, and dietary fiber.
TIP: Try adding cayenne pepper to meat and vegetable sauté, beans, salad dressing, and soups.

Chili Peppers:
With a name derived from the Latin *capsicum*, these fiery peppers are available throughout the year to add heat and spice to any dish. Better yet, chili peppers have many health benefits! They provide relief from the inflammation associated with arthritis, psoriasis, diabetic neuropathy, and osteoarthritis pain. They also help clear mucus from the respiratory tract and boost immunity with high levels of beta-carotene and vitamin A and C. In addition, chili peppers may help stop the spread of prostate cancer, reduce the risk of Type-2 diabetes, and prevent stomach ulcers. They are also a natural weight-loss aid.
TIP: If you can handle the heat, try adding habanera, chipotle, jalapeno, Anaheim, ancho, or Serrano peppers to vegetable omelets, burritos, pasta, guacamole, salad dressing, soups, and sandwiches.

Cilantro and Coriander Seeds:
These flavorful spices are also available throughout the year in whole seeds or ground powder. Coriander seeds have been traditionally used by many cultures as anti-diabetic, anti-inflammatory, and cholesterol-regulating spices, rich in nutrients and phytonutrients. Specific nutrients in coriander seeds include dietary fiber, iron, magnesium, and manganese.
TIP: Try adding coriander to meat, poultry and vegetable sauté, fish, pasta, tacos, omelets, soups, sauces, and broth.

Cinnamon:
While most popular during the cold winter months, cinnamon is available throughout the year. The brown bark from the cinnamon tree is available in two forms: dried sticks and ground powder. Cinnamon is known for its anti-clotting, anti-microbial, and anti-inflammatory properties. It is sometimes used as a food preservative, and helps control blood sugar, boost brain function, improve colon health, and protect against heart disease. Cinnamon is rich in manganese, fiber, iron, and calcium.

TIP: Try adding cinnamon to lamb, sautéd vegtables, oatmeal, and yams. Try some in your coffee too!

Cloves:
The buds from the evergreen clove tree are also available throughout the year. Cloves and clove oil are a great source of manganese, fiber, vitamin C, calcium, and magnesium, and contain omega-3 fatty acids. Health studies link cloves to treatment of digestive tract cancers, joint inflammation, dentistry anesthetics, and anti-bacterial agents like sore throat sprays and mouthwashes.
TIP: Try adding cloves to sautéed vegetables, meats, fruit, beans, curries, soups, sauces, broth, and poaching liquid.

Cumin:
Available year-round, cumin may be purchased either whole or ground. This peppery spice has health benefits that include digestive aid, cancer prevention, increase in energy levels, and immune system strengthening. Cumin is also an excellent source of iron.
TIP: Try adding cumin to chili, beans, nuts, curries, meats, poultry, fish, vegetables, rice, and fruit.

Dill:
While dried dill is available year-round, fresh dill is only available during the summer and fall. Dill has a unique flavor with added health benefits, including protection against carcinogens and free radicals, regulation of bacteria, and prevention of bone loss. Dill is rich in calcium, fiber, iron, and magnesium.
TIP: Try adding dill to vegetables, fish, sandwiches, egg salad, potatoes, and omelets.

Mustard Seeds:
This pungent spice is available in three varieties: white mustard, black mustard, and brown mustard. These seeds have great health benefits, including protection against gastrointestinal cancer and anti-inflammatory properties. Mustard seeds are a good source of selenium, magnesium, iron, calcium, zinc, manganese, protein, niacin, fiber, and omega-3 fatty acids.
TIP: Try adding mustard seeds to chicken breast, fish, salad dressing, salad, brown rice, and sauces.

Oregano:
Available throughout the year and cultivated around the world, oregano is known for its strong aroma and flavor. Rich in nutrients, oregano is a good source of fiber, iron, manganese, calcium, vitamins A, C, and K, and omega-3 fatty acids. The health benefits of oregano include anti-bacterial and strong anti-oxidant properties.
TIP: Try adding oregano to foods like tacos, pasta, sautéed vegetables and mushrooms, omelets and frittatas, garlic bread, and salad dressing.

Peppermint:
This very flavorful greenish-purple spice is available throughout the year. With health benefits including the ability to soothe an upset stomach, help you breathe easier, fight cancer, and act as an anti-bacterial agent, it's no wonder that peppermint is so popular. Peppermint is a great source of manganese, Vitamins A, C, and B2, beta-carotene, fiber, folate, iron, magnesium, calcium, potassium, copper, and omega-3 fatty acids.
TIP: Try adding peppermint to yogurt, sautéed vegetables and eggplant, salad, soups, fruit salad, and tea.

Rosemary:
Rosemary is very popular because of its unique flavor, fragrance, and year-round availability. The health benefits of rosemary include stimulation of the immune system and circulation, improved digestion, anti-inflammatory properties, and improved concentration. Rosemary is rich in nutrients like fiber, iron, and calcium.
TIP: Try adding rosemary to chicken, lamb, pork, salmon, tuna, omelets, frittatas, sauce, breads, vegetables, and soups.

Sage:
Fresh, whole-dried, and powdered sage is available year-round. The health benefits of sage include anti-inflammatory, anti-oxidant, and memory-enhancement properties.
TIP: Try adding sage to beans, chicken, fish, omelets, frittatas, casseroles, stews, sauces, yogurt, vegetables, and soups.

Thyme:
This widely-used and fragrant spice is freshly available throughout the year. The health benefits associated with thyme include aiding in chest and respiratory problems, as well as anti-oxidant, bacteria and fungus-fighting properties. Nutrients in thyme include iron, manganese, calcium, and fiber.
TIP: Try adding thyme to foods like fish, beans, omelets, scrambled eggs, sauces, stock, stews, and soups.

Turmeric:

This popular spice comes from the root of *curcuma longa*, a perennial plant in the ginger family. Health benefits associated with turmeric include anti-inflammatory properties, which are helpful for treating inflammatory bowel disease and rheumatoid arthritis. Turmeric also helps cystic fibrosis sufferers, fights cancer, may reduce the risk of childhood leukemia, improves liver function, protects cardiovascular function, helps lower cholesterol, and may protect against Alzheimer's disease. The nutrients found in turmeric are manganese, iron, vitamin B6, fiber, and potassium.

TIP: Try adding turmeric to foods like egg salad, brown rice, sautéed vegetables, lentils, fruit, salad dressing, and especially curry sauces and soups.

Nutrition, Special Health Topics, and Final Thoughts

The MY DIVA DIET mission is to give you as much power as possible to lead a life of superior health and happiness in the body you've always wanted. Increasing your knowledge about nutrition can empower you to succeed.

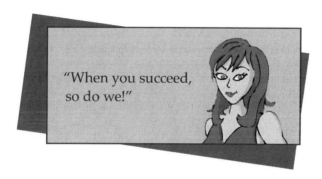

"When you succeed, so do we!"

MY DIVA DIET was designed from over twenty-five years of experience (via personal application and training clients) and education in the fitness industry, and it is backed up by sound nutrition. It's not a quick-fix solution, nor is it a gimmick offering false promises while your health actually declines. In fact, we have used nutrition as a main source in explaining and expanding on certain topics and in our guidelines, special designs, guides, tips, charts, meal options, and recipes.

Nutrition ✱

Nutrition is defined as the relationship between food and the health of the human body. When you achieve proper nutrition, all the essential nutrients are supplied and utilized in a balance that maintains optimal health and well-being. Good nutrition is essential for normal organ development and function, normal reproduction, growth, and maintenance, optimum activity level and working efficiency, resistance to infection and disease, and the ability to repair bodily damage or injury.

Balance is the basic principle of nutrition. The nutrition your body needs for health and exercise cannot be found in a single nutrient, but in a proper combination of all the essentials, including water, protein, carbohydrates, fats, vitamins, minerals, antioxidants, and other needed properties like fiber. These nutrients provide the foundation for building the body that you want, while allowing you to stay healthy in the process.

305

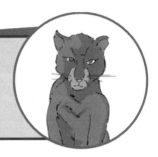

Consider taking a nutrition course or purchasing a book on nutrition. See our resources listed on page 308.

Here are some short definitions to help you build your nutritional vocabulary:

<u>Antioxidants</u> are molecules that can safely interact with free radicals and *terminate* the chain before healthy molecules are damaged. Vitamin E, beta-carotene, and vitamin C are powerful antioxidants. Fruits and vegetables are full of antioxidants.

<u>Carbohydrates</u> are the best source of energy for all bodily functions, especially the brain and central nervous system, and for muscle exertion. They also assist in the digestion and assimilation of foods. Carbohydrates are made up of the chemical elements carbon, hydrogen, and oxygen, which provide us with immediate and long term energy. Carbohydrates also help regulate protein and fat metabolism.

<u>Carotenoids</u> are antioxidants that work to destroy free-radical and damage-causing disease agents. They are found in dark orange, red, yellow, and green fruits and vegetables.

<u>Cholesterol</u> is a fatty substance (lipid) produced by the liver and required for good cellular health. If you have too much cholesterol in your blood, it sticks to your arterial walls. This buildup is called plaque, and it can narrow your arterial passages or even block them completely. High levels of cholesterol in the blood can increase the risk of heart disease. Since the body makes its own cholesterol, dietary needs are low. High-cholesterol foods are mainly found in animal products like egg yolks, meat, poultry, seafood, and high-fat dairy products.

<u>Fats–or lipids</u> are the most concentrated source of energy in the diet. There are three classes of lipids: triglycerides, phospholipids, and sterols. There are three "essential" fatty acids that cannot be made from the breakdown of other substances in the body and must be supplied by the diet: linoleic, linolenic, and arachidonic acids. These polyunsaturated fats are necessary for normal growth and for healthy blood, arteries,

and nerves. In addition to supplying energy and providing valuable nutrients to the body, fats act as carriers for fat-soluble vitamins. Natural oils also nourish the skin and scalp.

Fiber is the indigestible substance that is found in the outer layers of plants (grains, fruits, vegetables, legumes, and nuts) that aid digestion and clean out the intestines (see more on fiber in this section).

Free Radicals are groups of atoms that form when oxygen interacts with certain molecules. When they react with important cellular components like DNA or cell membranes, they can impair cell function or kill cells entirely. The body uses antioxidants to prevent free radical damage.

Macronutrients are nutrients that provide calories (energy). Nutrients are substances needed for growth, metabolism, and other body functions. Since "macro" means large, macronutrients are needed in large amounts. Macronutrients in the diet that are the key sources of energy are namely protein, carbohydrates, and fat.

Micronutrients are certain vitamins or minerals (iodine, vitamin A, iron, zinc, and folate) that are only needed in minute amounts. They play a role in the production of enzymes, hormones and other substances, helping to regulate growth, activity, development and functioning of the immune and reproductive systems.

Minerals are essential nutrients the human body needs in small amounts to work properly. They are necessary for building strong bones and teeth, controlling fluids inside and outside cells, turning the food we eat into energy. They also help with blood glucose levels, regulate heartbeat and blood pressure, and much more. Minerals can be found in most plant foods (whole grains, nuts, fruits, and vegetables), seafood, and some animal protein.

Phytochemicals are chemical substances that act like antioxidants and are found in fruits and vegetables. Phytochemicals appear to block the processes that lead to cancer, and it's possible that they reduce tumor formation.

Phytoestrogens are compounds found in plants that work like a weak form of estrogen. They may create an environment that helps prevent hormonally-linked types of cancer from forming, including breast and prostate cancer. They may also help reduce the risk of cardiovascular disease, provide protection against osteoporosis, and alleviate menopausal symptoms. Foods that are high in phytoestrogens are flax seed, soybeans, and tofu. Other plant foods contain smaller amounts.

Polyphenols are antioxidant compounds found in fruits and vegetables that help prevent cancer and heart disease. While polyphenols are found widely in plants (whether in roots, leaves, fruits or vegetables), the best sources are in green and black tea, wine, onions, apples, strawberries, nuts, and yams.

Protein is an essential nutrient. "Next to water, protein is the most plentiful substance in the human body." It is critical for the maintenance of good health and growth and development of all body components. All tissues, bones, and nerves are made up of protein. It is the main building material for muscles, blood, skin, hair, nails, and internal organs, including the heart and brain.

Vitamins are organic food substances that regulate the functioning of our bodies and cells, and they are found only in plants and animals. The body cannot make its own vitamins; they must be supplied via diet or supplements. There are two main categories of vitamins: water-soluble (B-complex, vitamin C, and bioflavonoids) and fat-soluble (A,D, E, and K).

✻ Nutrition Resources:
- Nutrition Almanac Fourth Edition, by Gayla J. Kirschmann and John D. Kirschmann (1996)
- The Tufts University Guide to Total Nutrition, by Stanley Gershoff, PH.D. Dean Emeritus of the Tufts University School of Nutrition (1996)

Special Health Topics
FYI: Honey, Agave Nectar, Molasses, and Sugar:

Honey is a sweet, thick, sugary substance produced by bees and derived from the nectar of flowers. It consists of varying proportions of fructose, glucose, water, oil, and special enzymes produced by bees. Honey also contains trace amounts of vitamins and minerals, and tiny amounts of compounds that may function as antioxidants.

Agave nectar (syrup) is a plant-based sweetener derived from a cactus native to Mexico. It has been used for centuries to make tequila. Agave nectar is primarily fructose and glucose. It is very sweet and light, with only twenty calories per teaspoon, and it is very low on the glycemic index.

Molasses, a thick, brown to deep black honey-like substance, is produced when cane or beet sugar is processed. It contains approximately the same amount of calories as sugar, but only about half the sucrose. It consists of both glucose and fructose.

Dietary sugar is primarily comprised of refined sugar cane or sugar beet. Table sugar (granulated white sugar) is pure sucrose and is stripped of all vitamins, minerals, fiber, amino acids, and trace elements during the refinement process. To learn more about sugar see our Food Additives section in PART SIX.

Fiber: The Abandoned Substance
The American diet is full of processed and man-made food products. These foods rarely, if ever, contain fiber. To make matters worse, it's relatively rare to see fresh and natural legumes, nuts, seeds, whole grains, vegetables, and fruits on an American table. With this kind of diet there will be consequences!

What is constipation?
Constipation commonly means infrequent bowel movements, difficulty during defecation, and incomplete bowel evacuation.

What are the causes of constipation?
- Lack of daily fiber in the diet
- Dehydration
- Lack of physical activity
- Too much milk and other dairy products, like cheese
- Medications
- Irritable bowel syndrome
- Life changes or routine fluctuations such as pregnancy, aging, and travel
- Abuse of laxatives
- Ignoring the urge to have a bowel movement
- Specific diseases
- Problems with the colon and rectum
- Problems with intestinal function

What about fiber supplements?

Considering the lack of fiber in the American diet, it is no wonder that companies have developed strategies to capitalize on this related problem. We eat so much sugar, flour, beef, and too many packaged, processed, and man-made foods. We consume excessive amounts of alcohol and medications (and drugs) and then we wonder why we are constipated. In response to our outcry, we are inundated with "poop" powders, pills, and potions. We don't have to eat raw fruits, vegetables, nuts, and legumes–we can just take a pill and then have a bowel movement! But did you know that the frequency, texture and color of your bowel movement provide a lot of information about your diet and health?

- An occasional powder or pill to help with bowel regularity may be okay–just make sure its content is not synthetic.
- Moderate your intake of natural laxatives–they can cause bloating and become addictive.
- Occasional colon cleansing is a great idea–just make sure the product or program is safe and healthy!

> "Where's the water and fiber? The American diet lacks water and fibrous foods, so we become dehydrated and constipated–two unhealthy conditions that can leave you miserable."

Fiber

Fiber is necessary for proper digestion and elimination. The key health benefit of fiber is its regulation of intestinal track function, and a high-fiber diet may prevent common intestinal ailments like constipation, hemorrhoids, and diverticulosis. Fiber has also been linked to the prevention of colon and breast cancer. In addition, fiber can help lower blood sugar and manage diabetes and obesity.

Types of Fiber:

Soluble and insoluble fiber are not actually digested as they travel through the digestive system. This means that instead of being absorbed into the bloodstream for use as energy, fiber excretes from the body. Soluble fiber is broken down in digestion and creates a jelly-like mass around digested food. This helps bowel regularity and lowers cholesterol. Insoluble fiber is not broken down during digestion and therefore works as an "intestinal scrubber", helping prevent constipation. Recommended fiber consumption is 25 to 35 grams per day. Sources of fiber include legumes, nuts, seeds, grain, fruits, and vegetables.

> Protect your colon–it is the place from which many diseases start. Increase your intake of fibrous foods and water! You will be happier, healthier, and leaner.

Top Fibrous Foods

Legumes

1.	Cowpeas:	½ cup	= 8.3 grams of fiber
2.	Chick peas:	½ cup	= 7 grams of fiber
3.	Kidney beans:	½ cup	= 6.9 grams of fiber
4.	Lima beans:	½ cup	= 6.8 grams of fiber
5.	Navy beans:	½ cup	= 4.9 grams of fiber

Grains

1.	Triticale:	½ cup raw	= 8.7 grams of fiber
2.	Bran (corn):	2 Tbsp. raw	= 7.9 grams of fiber
3.	Amaranth seeds:	¼ cup raw	= 7.5 grams of fiber
4.	Rye:	¼ cup raw	= 6.2 grams of fiber
5.	Barley:	½ cup cooked	= 4.4 grams of fiber

Hot Cereal

1.	Raiston:	¾ cup cooked	= 6 grams of fiber
2.	Wheatena:	¾ cup cooked	= 4 grams of fiber
3.	Quaker oatmeal:	½ cup dry	= 4 grams of fiber
4.	Quinoa Inca Red:	¼ cup dry	= 4 grams of fiber
5.	Lundberg Cream of Rice:	¼ cup dry	= 3 grams of fiber

Nuts & Seeds

1.	Pine nuts (dried):	1 oz.	= 4.1 grams of fiber
2.	Pumpkin seeds (dried):	1 oz. hulled	= 3.9 grams of fiber
3.	Chestnuts (roasted):	1 oz.	= 3.7 grams of fiber
4.	Pistachios (dried):	1 oz.	= 3.1 grams of fiber
5.	Coconut (raw):	1 oz. grated	= 2.5 grams of fiber

Fruits
1.	Cherimoya:	½ (10 oz.)	= 8.7 grams of fiber
2.	Blackberries:	1 cup	= 7.2 grams of fiber
3.	Guava:	1 (3 oz.)	= 4.9 grams of fiber
4.	Pear:	1 serving	= 4.3 grams of fiber
5.	Breadfruit:	1 (3 oz.)	= 4.2 grams of fiber

Vegetables
1.	Artichoke Hearts:	½ cup (boiled)	= 4.4 grams of fiber
2.	Bamboo Shoots:	1 cup (sliced)	= 3.9 grams of fiber
3.	Parsnips:	½ cup (sliced, boiled)	= 3.8 grams of fiber
4.	Chicory:	½ cup (chopped, raw)	= 3.6 grams of fiber ·
5.	Pumpkin (canned):	½ cup	= 3.4 grams of fiber

Probiotics

The human body has both good and bad bacteria, and some are good for health. The lining in the gut and digestive processes do not function correctly without good bacteria, known as probiotics (meaning *for life*). This friendly bacteria balances the bodies internal environment and are essential to health in many ways: they enhance function of the gastrointestinal tract; protect against harmful pathogenic (disease causing) bacteria, viruses, fungi, and parasites; maintain the chemical (pH) of the digestive system; contribute to the assimilation of nutrients and elimination of toxins; and are critical to the immune system.

In a healthy state, our bodies naturally maintain the proper balance. However, there are things that disrupt this balance, including preservatives and additives in food, diets with a very high fat content, birth control pills, antibiotics and other medications (and drugs), caffeine and alcohol consumption, and even stress.

Sources of probiotics:

Yogurt is a great source for probiotics, but some yogurts don't actually contain "live bacteria" due to processing and high sugar content. Yogurts with live bacteria contain *Lactobacillus bulgaricus* and *Streptococcus thermophilus*. Look for yogurts that *contain* (not made with) "live and active cultures". Other sources include aged cheese, kefir, cultured dairy products, and fermented foods (pickles, sauerkraut, kimchi, miso).

Another way to make sure get sufficient amounts of probiotics is to supplement with acidophilus. Acidophilus can suppress Candida and prevent diarrhea and constipation. It helps reduce gas, bloating, and bad breath, and counteract lactose intolerance. It may also enhance immune system function, aid in the treatment of respiratory infections like sinusitis and bronchitis, and lower the risk of developing asthma.

Seafood and Pork: Addressing the Confusion *

Eating meat and seafood seems to be a confusing topic of debate in the world of dieting. Eat meat; don't eat meat? Eat shrimp; don't eat shrimp? Pork: is it really the other white meat?

Seafood:

Most shellfish, and some other fish, are basically the scavengers of the ocean (or as Dr. Don Colbert calls them: "the cockroaches of the sea"). They act as natural cleansing agents in the sea (the same way the pool cleaner skims the debris and algae from your swimming pool), so they are full of pollutants. These pollutants don't necessarily make the shellfish sick, but they are passed on to humans when the shellfish are eaten.

Because of this, MY DIVA DIET recommend eating "clean fish" with fins, and avoiding the following: catfish, clams, crabs, crayfish, European flat fish, lobster, lump-fish, monkfish, mussels, oysters, prawns, scallops, sculpins, shark, shrimp, sturgeon, swordfish. Also avoid raw fish, as they may contain parasites that are otherwise killed in cooking.

The Dark Side of Pork:

You may know pork as "the other white meat". But there are some facts about pork meat to consider when deciding whether or not to incorporate it into your diet. First, pigs eat large quantities of food, which dilutes the hydrochloric acid concentration in their stomachs. This allows toxins, viruses, parasites, and bacteria to invade their flesh, which may be present when we eat the meat. Pigs are similar to shellfish, in that they cleanse the earth of its toxic material–they will eat anything!

Also consider that 1 slice of bacon has around 21 grams of fat; 3.5 ounces of ham has 11 grams of fat; 1 pork chop has around 6 grams of fat; 6 spare ribs have 35 grams of fat; and all are high in cholesterol.

‾
* Resource on Seafood and Pork:
- Don Colbert, M.D., board certified family practitioner and author of What Would Jesus Eat, Walking in Divine Health, The Bible Cure Series, and The Seven Pillars of Health.

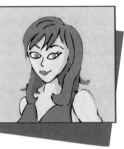

"Whatever a living creature has eaten will end up in its meat— thus if we eat it, we are exposed to any toxins it may have."

Additives, Preservatives, Pesticides, Herbicides, Antibiotics, Hormones, and Animal Cruelty... the American Way

We find ourselves in the Age of "Instant Gratification", where we have everything within minutes, even if it is not good for us. The internet provides immediate information, regardless of its accuracy. "YouTube" and "Reality TV" offers on-the-spot entertainment even at the expense of our morality and dignity. Fitness and beauty is created in seconds, often without any discipline. Money is no different: just look at the success of the state lottery system; people are willing to spend their last dollar on luck. And the medical field also promises instant satisfaction–just take a pill and your ailment will go away! Even marketing agencies are in on it (or is it the pharmaceutical companies?). They make everyone look so happy while they spout a laundry list of side effects–nausea, vomiting, headache, nosebleeds, dry mouth, heart palpitations, etc.!

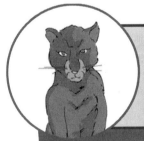

Consider this warning: If you experience death after you take this medication, call your doctor immediately!

The food industry is no exception. Americans want their food and they want it fast no matter how it is made. So manufacturers continue to accommodate this desire. Desire is the key word–we *need* food to live, but we *desire* convenient, tasty, cheap food. But we should realize that food that is poorly grown, made, and manufactured (whether processed, packaged, man-made, or via animal cruelty–hormones, antibiotics, living conditions and their death) is *not* cheap. We pay for it in other ways: poor health, obesity, premature death, environmental problems, brutality toward innocent animals, and the corruption of government and large corporations. But who is really to blame here? Is it the companies that make the products to increase their bottom line, or are we culpable for buying into the machine?

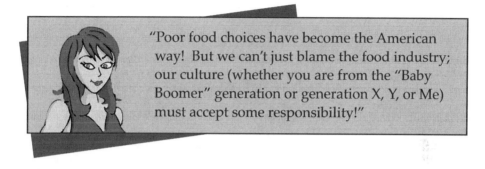

"Poor food choices have become the American way! But we can't just blame the food industry; our culture (whether you are from the "Baby Boomer" generation or generation X, Y, or Me) must accept some responsibility!"

Processed Foods

According to many fitness and health professionals, about 90% of Americans' food budget are used to buy processed foods. Gone are the days when wholesome foods in their natural form were the main staple of the American diet. Food products have taken that place–and we wonder why we are over-weight and unhealthy.

- Fresh fruits? No way–just have a fruit roll-up or a fruit cup.
- Fresh cut of halibut–what is that? Let's have some frozen, fried, battered fish sticks instead.
- Fresh filet mignon is replaced by frozen dinners.
- Turkey breast is replaced with lunchmeat or sausage.
- Potatoes become potato chips or French fries.
- Oats or other whole grains are processed into sugary cereals, white bread, crackers, cakes, and cookies.
- Fresh asparagus is replaced by slimy spikes in a green can.
- Wholesome foods are combined with countless other ingredients, the first of which is sugar and the rest of which we can't pronounce.
- Produce is contaminated with pesticides, herbicides, and other harmful by-products of the production process, ruining what nature had intended for health and energy.

Originally additives and preservatives were created to increase the shelf life of foods, to enhance or manipulate flavor, and at times to add nutrients for certain vitamin deficiencies. At a time when food was scarce, this idea had some merit. Somewhere along the way, though, someone forgot the original purpose and began to over-produce these foods with no regard for the unnecessary (and in some cases unsafe) preservatives and additives used or the effect it would have on human health.

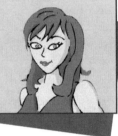

"Humans were meant to be stewards over animals, but today we have truly abused that privilege. There is nothing worse than intentional misuse of power and authority. Americans have lost their consciences and replaced them with greed and gluttony, made worse by laziness."

Food from Animals

Here are some things to think about when considering eating beef, poultry, and fish:

#1 Cattle are raised in deplorable conditions and horrifically slaughtered. And while dairy farms may not kill their animals, they do inject their cows with hormones and antibiotics with no regard for the cow or the quality of the product they are making.

#2 The plight of chickens is no better than that of cows. Chickens are often debeaked and stuffed into cramped cages, where they are forced to live out their lives never experiencing freedom. Their feet grow into and around the bottoms of their wire cages, instead of scratching in the dirt and looking for food the way free-range chickens do. Are they killed any more humanely than the cows?

#3 There are also "farm-raised" fish! Do they get a break? Can the fish "farmers" possibly emulate the natural environment to which the fish have adapted over time, or provide for the needs of the fish as well as nature would? What about pollutants and other harmful factors? And, are our fishing methods humane? When a proud or less-experienced fisherman wants a photograph before he "catches and releases", does the fish suffer?

#4   The way an animal is raised is not the only factor affecting the meat on the tables of millions of Americans. Mass-produced cattle, chickens, and pigs are not being fed quality food. Some are able to exercise and feed on grass, but most live in close, cramped environments and when food supplies run low they are forced to eat their own manure, and sometimes even their own young.

#5   The method of slaughter, if done improperly, distresses the animal and can affect the meat you eat. This phenomenon is called *"fight or flight"*, and it involves the response that occurs in moments of genuine fear. True animal lovers can empathize with this idea. The adrenaline produced by the animal during its final moments of fear actually ends up in the blood stream, affecting the meat.

#6   STOP for a moment to consider Mad Cow Disease, Bird Flu, mercury poisoning, and other foodborne diseases.

#7   Even after earning hundreds of thousands of dollars for their owners, American champion racehorses that can no longer race or win are sold to slaughter houses at rock-bottom prices. These former athletes are sold to the "meat man", then sent off to a "livestock auction" and to their final destination, a "kill pen". They are killed, sometimes more inhumanely than cows and chickens, and then shipped to Japan and Europe as food for human consumption or as pet food.

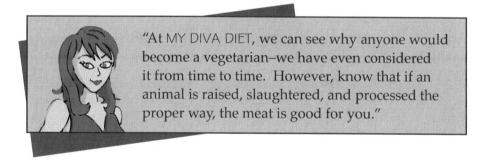

"At MY DIVA DIET, we can see why anyone would become a vegetarian—we have even considered it from time to time. However, know that if an animal is raised, slaughtered, and processed the proper way, the meat is good for you."

Facts on Kosher Rules and Slaughtering:
- Do not eat animals that die of natural causes or are killed by other animals.
- Do not eat animals with evidence of disease or flaws in the organs at the time of slaughter.

- The ritual of the slaughter is known as *shechitah*, and the person who performs the slaughter is called a *shochet* (meaning to destroy or kill).
- The method of slaughter is painless, causes unconsciousness within seconds, and is widely recognized as the most humane method of slaughter.
- Another advantage of *shechitah* is that it ensures rapid, complete drainage of blood, which is necessary to render the meat kosher.

Look for the Kosher Triangle:

The Kosher triangle is a trademark that signifies *"kashruth"* (kosher). The triangle is a symbol of integrity representing the most trusted and reliable name in strict rabbinical food certification and supervision. It is great to know that the products that earn this symbol are governed by strict laws. Kosher operations must pass a thorough investigation of their facility, procedures, equipment, ingredients, and processes used in the production of a food product. Each food product must be inspected and certified separately. The certification process is ongoing; each product must be inspected every year.

Facts on Wild vs. Farm-Raised Fish:

Not only do farm-raised fish lack the health benefits of wild fish, but they are also more likely to get sick. Farm-raised fish are fed concentrated protein pellets instead of their natural diet. This feed seems to contaminate the fish, and they contain higher levels of toxins (PCBs, dioxin, etc.) than wild fish. Farm-raised fish are also fatter, and these chemicals are stored in the fatty tissue. Some farm-raised fish are processed inhumanely. First, they are sedated with clove oil that is poured into the water. Then, carbon dioxide is added until their brain functions cease but their hearts continue to beat. Finally, their gills are cut so they bleed out and they are gilled, gutted, and then processed.

Facts on Free-Range Livestock (cage-free cattle, pigs and poultry):

Free-range means that the animals are able to move and feed at will, not confined in a battery or a pen. Whether poultry, eggs, or beef, free-range livestock should meet these criteria:

- No antibiotics
- No hormones
- No pesticides or herbicides used in the soil or feed
- No artificial ingredients

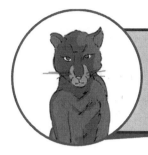

A healthier, happier cow, turkey, chicken, or fish means healthier food for humans!

Other Facts on Organic Foods and Free-range Foods:

Free-range beef has a lower overall fat content because the cattle exercise. They are also free of pesticides, herbicides from their feedlot, antibiotics, and hormones. Organic, free-range chickens are raised primarily on grains and grasses, and are kept free of hormones, antibiotics, pesticides, and herbicides. They are significantly lower in fat than chickens raised in "chicken factories", and also produce eggs with higher nutritional value.

Facts on Organic Foods:

Organic foods are produced according to certain standards. Organic crops are grown without the use of conventional pesticides, herbicides, artificial fertilizers, human waste, or sewage sludge, and they are processed without ionizing radiation or food additives. Organically-raised animals are reared without routine use of antibiotics or growth hormones. An organic product must not be genetically modified.

Is Organic Food Really Better? *

Not only do you eliminate harmful chemicals by consuming organic foods but, according to research done on organic foods, you get a more nutritious food. Consider these studies:

Study #1: The recent $25-milllion (the largest of its kind) study done by a European Union-funded project
Findings: "Organically produced crops and dairy milk contain more beneficial compounds–such as vitamins and antioxidants".

Study #2: 2003 study in Journal of Agricultural Food Chemistry
Findings: "Fruits and vegetables grown organically show significantly higher levels of cancer-fighting antioxidants than conventionally grown foods".

Study #3: U.S. research team from Emory University in Atlanta
Findings: After analyzing urine samples from children ages three to eleven who ate only organic foods they found that "they contained virtually no metabolites of two common pesticides, malathion and chlorpyrifos. However, once the children returned to eating conventionally grown foods, concentrations of these pesticides quickly climbed to 263 parts per billion, says the study."

Study #4: The Food Commission in Britain
Findings: Analysis of government nutrition data (from the 1930s and 2002) on meat and dairy products found that "the mineral content of milk, cheese, and beef declined as much as 70 percent".

✱ Resources on Organic Food Studies
• Times Online, "Eat Your Words, All Who Scoff at Organic Food", by Jon Ungoed-Thomas (October 28, 2007).
• Science Daily, "Organically Grown Foods Higher In Cancer-fighting Chemicals Than Conventionally Grown Foods" (March 4, 2003).
• Common Dreams.Org News Center, "New Studies Back Benefits of Organic Diet", by Stephen Leahy (March 4, 2006)

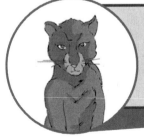

Following are a few other websites and articles you can get information about organic foods and their overall benefits.

#1 – The Organic Center *www.organic-center.org*
State of Science Review: Nutritional Superiority of Organic Foods
"New Evidence Confirms the Nutritional Superiority of Plant-based Organic Foods", by Charles Benbrook, Xin Zhao, Jaime Yanez, Neal Davies and Preston Andrew (March 2008)

#2 – Organic Consumer Association–*www.organicconsumers.org*
"Is Organic Food More Nutritious?", by Marian Burros,
The New York Times (July 2003)

#3 – Earth Future Earth - *www.earthfuture.com/earth*
"Ten Reasons Why Organic Food is Better", by Guy Dauncey (August 2002)

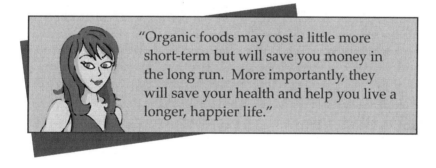

"Organic foods may cost a little more short-term but will save you money in the long run. More importantly, they will save your health and help you live a longer, happier life."

Food Labeling–Truth * Health * Safety:

The U.S. Department of Agriculture (USDA) regulates meat and the Food and Drug Administration (FDA) regulates all other food. Are we supposed to trust the FDA, USDA, and food companies to help ensure that our food supplies are safe, healthy, and truthfully represented and labeled? Yes and No!

There are restrictions when it comes to the labeling of foods but there are plenty of gaps. It has become an extremely complex problem and can be confusing and misleading. Here are just a couple of examples:

Natural:
According the USDA, food can only be labeled "natural" if it contains no artificial ingredients or added colors and is minimally processed. Animal products raised with the use of artificial hormones and genetically modified foods, *can* be labeled "natural". Also it is important to note that "natural" does not mean organic.

Organic:
To be certified organic, companies must not allow the use of hormones, antibiotics, synthetic fertilizers, bioengineering, and radiation. However, the way an animal is treated (or slaughtered) and other environmental concerns do not apply to the guidelines (or the enforcement) of being certified organic and the USDA rules do not fully address these concerns.

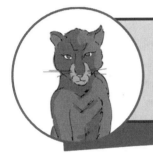

This is why we go the extra step–BUY KOSHER whenever possible–especially when it comes to foods from animal sources!

Who's watching your back (butt)? It's probably the guy at the supermarket, bus stop, auto repair shop, gym, or school. But when it comes to "food health and safety" don't count solely on the government or the food companies! Be vigilant and do your own research!

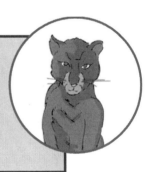

Final Thoughts:
Contrary to what some would have you believe, most additives and preservatives, pesticides (and other chemicals), or any food derived from cruelly-treated animals are not healthy or safe. We really don't even know the extent of the damage caused by foods and food products made this way. So many choices and variables exist that it seems impossible to test whether a product is safe or unsafe until it's too late. It's easy to blame genetics or other abstract factors, but someday we will put all the pieces together and finally discover: "We are what we eat–whether good or bad!"

"Our modern society today lacks knowledge and compassion. No longer do we strive for what is right; instead, we look the other way. Let's change OUR AMERICAN WAY and take care of our bodies, our environment, our children, and our innocent animals. Let's become more informed and health-conscious. Let's escape greed, gluttony, and laziness. Let's tap into our compassionate and courageous sides and work to implement humane and safe methods within our food industry!"

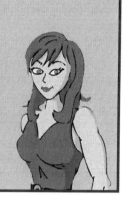

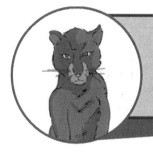

There are real steps we all can take to help now: choose clean and pure foods. Choose food that is natural, fresh, organic, and kosher. Choose clean, healthy, fibrous and *alive* foods!

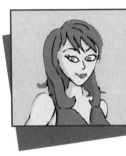

"We can also subscribe to the MY DIVA DIET way of life and/or begin a diet program that gives us the truth, steers us toward a lifestyle of proper eating and exercise, and encourages accountability and discipline!"

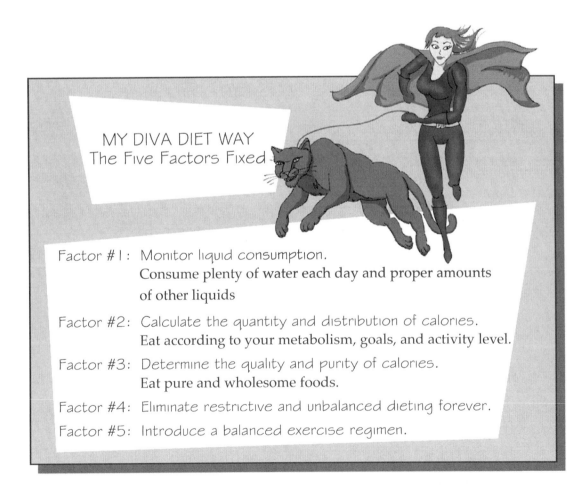

MY DIVA DIET WAY
The Five Factors Fixed

Factor #1: Monitor liquid consumption.
Consume plenty of water each day and proper amounts of other liquids

Factor #2: Calculate the quantity and distribution of calories.
Eat according to your metabolism, goals, and activity level.

Factor #3: Determine the quality and purity of calories.
Eat pure and wholesome foods.

Factor #4: Eliminate restrictive and unbalanced dieting forever.

Factor #5: Introduce a balanced exercise regimen.

PART EIGHT

My Workspace

We can do anything we want if we stick to it long enough.
~ Helen Keller

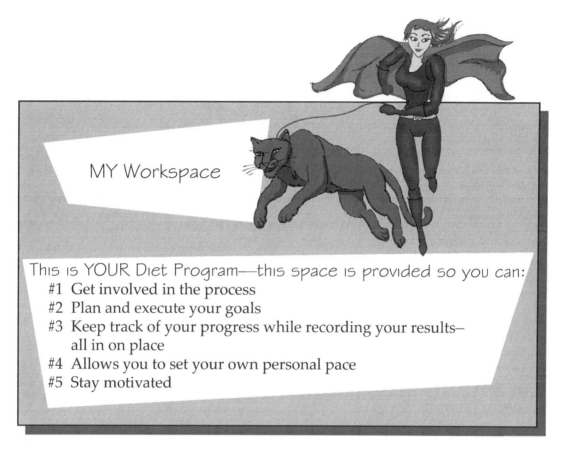

MY Workspace

This is YOUR Diet Program—this space is provided so you can:
- #1 Get involved in the process
- #2 Plan and execute your goals
- #3 Keep track of your progress while recording your results— all in on place
- #4 Allows you to set your own personal pace
- #5 Stay motivated

Introduction to Eight Diva Worksheets

Diva Worksheet #1:

MY DIVA DIET Simple Summary for Fat Loss (Phase One—Diva Reduction)
This worksheet allows you to view MY DIVA DIET for losing fat (while improving health) at a glance and provides you with a place to make notes on your diet and other related concerns.

MY DIVA DIET Society Guide
This section provides some tips that focus directly on different types of women (or young girls) and addresses their specific concerns about dieting and exercise.

Diva Worksheet #2:

Diva Diet Quiz Summary—The Five Factors Scores and Diet Villains Exposed
Use this worksheet to summarize your diet quiz from PART THREE (pages 61-83):

- Score your total diet and exercise program and make notes on potential solutions
- Score your Five Factors and discover your problem areas
- Expose your personal Diet Villains

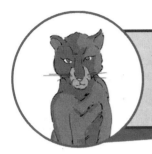

You can take the Diva Diet Quiz periodically. This will make it easier for you stay up-to-date on the changes in your diet and exercise habits—and help keep you on track.

Diva Worksheet #3
3-Day Diet Analysis Instructions and Food Diary Sheets
Use the food diary sheets to write down everything you eat and drink for at least three days. When you're finished, follow the instructions provided so you can get a better picture of your daily eating habits, total calories, and nutrient breakdowns.

Diva Worksheet #4
3-Day Diet Analysis Totals:
Daily Calories and Nutrient Totals—Nutrient Ratio Calculations
Use this worksheet to record your 3-Day Diet Analysis totals. You can then calculate your daily nutrient ratio by following the Paw Guides provided.

Diva Worksheet #5
Personal Goals: Instructions and MY DIVA DIET Goal Sheet
Setting goals, both long-term and short-term, is a great way to begin your journey toward getting healthy & fit. Use this worksheet as a reality check that can get you started, and keep you going.

Body Composition Information
It is very important to understand the difference between weight loss and fat loss. Know how to determine your initial body fat so you can set realistic goals and differentiate between actual weight loss and fat loss as you move forward down your path of a great body and superior health.

Diva Worksheet #6
Progress Report

Tracking your progress can be a fun and valuable part of the journey toward losing fat and gaining health. Use this worksheet to track body weight and body fat, measurements, clothing size, and medical conditions.

Note on weighing yourself: Once you have obtained your initial numbers and calculated your fat-loss goals in pounds, inches, and size in clothes, write them down. Make sure you only weigh yourself once per week and at the same time of day. Use the same scale under the same conditions each time (for example, in the morning on an empty stomach rather than after a late dinner party). Maintaining a once-per-week weigh-in schedule is important to sustaining a positive state of mind. Women normally fluctuate five pounds depending on sodium intake, food intake, water balance, alcohol consumption, hormones, and medications (and drugs), so constantly monitoring all these insignificant fluctuations can impede your motivation.

Note on tracking your progress: Record your body composition and measurements every two weeks, beginning with week four. This will help gauge your progress and keep you on track, and you can use this information to make any necessary adjustments along the way. After your tenth week on MY DIVA DIET, make a final Progress Report to see how far you've come! If you have reached your goals at this time, continue to monitor and measure your body fat and measurements every three to four months to make sure you maintain your hard-earned results.

Diva Worksheet #7
3-Week Diet and Exercise Calendar

Use this calendar to track your weekly body weight. You can rate your overall eating habits, track your total calories, and indicate your "cheat days". You can also keep a record of your daily exercise. This is a great tool to monitor your daily performance and give you a weekly summary of your overall diet and exercise program! You'll stay focused because you can adjust your habits as needed along the way.

Diva Worksheet #8
MY DIVA DIET Journal

Use this area to write down your feelings about dieting, your body fat, or anything else you deem necessary. This can be your secret space, like a diary, or you can use it to write down concerns, questions or comments. You can also use this space for your grocery shopping lists and recipes you want to try.

Thank you for trusting MY DIVA DIET. Because our success depends on yours we have provided you with all the tools and information you will need to lose unwanted pounds, firm your body, entirely transform your physique, gain or regain your health, prevent obesity and poor health, or simply discover healthier lifestyle habits.

We are here for you throughout your journey, from the initial stages of setting your goals and performing a proper analysis to the end of your expedition. We are here for you if you hit a plateau or have questions. We can help you examine and figure out where to make adjustments so you can continue successfully on your path toward fat loss and improved health.

Our mission is to help you obtain or even exceed your goals. We want to hear all about your progress and help you celebrate your victories! We want you to be part of OUR story—helping women of all ages get healthy & fit.

Sincerely, MS Diva and Paw
www.MyDivaDiet.com

Diva Worksheet #1
MY DIVA DIET Simple Summary for Fat Loss
(Phase One—Diva Reduction)

This section provides you with a condensed version of MY DIVA DIET (Phase One— Diva Reduction). You can use this space for notes on:

- The Five Factors (PART ONE)
- The Diet Villains (PART ONE)
- The Diet (PART TWO)
- The Guidelines (PART FOUR)

By completing this worksheet, you can maintain an updated quick-reference guide to relevant topics without the necessity of referring to the book itself. This is just a summary – the full diet directions can be found in PART TWO—The Diet, while more in-depth guidelines are found in PART FOUR—The Guidelines.

Phase One—Diva Reduction
Focus on reduction for a ten-week period, or until you attain your fat-loss and health goals.

Phase One Cheating
Limit to once per week, choosing from the Diva Smart Diet Cheat Sheet (pages 216-219).

Factor #1: Liquid Consumption (Quiz # 1-8)

#1 Water
Ample water consumption (approximately 8-10 cups) throughout each day.

#2 Coffee and other caffeinated drinks
Moderate coffee consumption is okay. Just avoid excess fat and sugar normally used in coffee and coffee drinks. Limit your intake of other high caffeinated liquids like "energy drinks".

#3 Tea
Tea consumption is great if it is plain so don't be tempted to add sugar and/or cream. Stay clear of pre-made teas unless they are plain.

#4 Soda
Avoid soda of all kinds.

331

#5 Other drinks

Avoid sugar-filled drinks such as sport drinks, powdered soft drinks, juice boxes, and others.

#6 Juice

Limit juice consumption to freshly-squeezed only.

#7 Meal-replacement drinks

Limit your consumption of protein shakes, smoothies, green and other veggie drinks to those with superior nutritional content and those that are low in sugar and other unneeded additives.

#8 Alcohol

Avoid alcohol during this phase to achieve desired results more quickly.

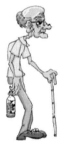
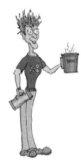
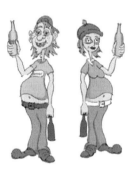

POPS   **CAFF**   **AL AND COLE**

FOLLOWING THESE LIQUID CONSUMPTION GUIDELINES WILL ENSURE FAT LOSS AND BETTER HEALTH—AND YOU WON'T BE DEHYDRATED, HYPER, ADDICTED, AND BAFFLED LIKE POPS, CAFF, AL, AND COLE!

Notes For Factor #1:

Factor #2: Quantity And Distribution of Calories (Quiz # 9–13)

#9 Daily Caloric Intake

Maintain 1,200-1,300 calories per day.

* More if you know you can lose fat on higher calories.

#10 Daily Nutrient Ratio 35-45-20

This ratio means that 35% of your daily calories should come from protein sources, 45% from carbohydrates, and 20% from fats.

* On a 1,300 calorie day, this equals 113.8 grams of protein, 146.3 grams of carbohydrates, and 28.9 grams of fat.

#11 Number of Meals per Day

Eat four small meals evenly spaced throughout the day (five is okay) to allow calories to be used for their intended purpose: health and energy.

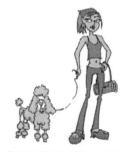

**GIRLIE DIE AND
HER POODLE, IT**

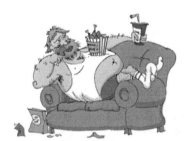

JOE STUFFT

OVEREATING LIKE JOE STUFT WILL ONLY DRAIN YOUR ENERGY, CAUSING WEIGHT GAIN AND LAZINESS! LIKEWISE, IF YOU UNDER-EAT LIKE GIRLIE DIE WITH HER POODLE IT, YOUR STARVING WILL LEAD TO LACK OF ENERGY AND MANY SHORT-AND LONG-TERM HEALTH ISSUES.

#12 Meal Timing

Eat frequent small meals at regular intervals throughout the day.

* Schedule three to four hours between meals, consuming larger meals in the morning or afternoon.
* Dinner portions should be smaller, consisting of lean protein and vegetables.
* If you get hungry between meals, fix a small, nutritious snack.

#13   Meal Size (portion control)
        Control your portions at each meal.
        • Try to distribute your 1,300 calories between four meals, at approximately
          325 calories per meal.
        • For more help on portion control see the Paw Guide below and in PART
          FOUR (pages 103-107):

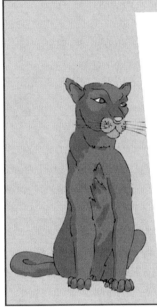

Paw Portion Guide

• Protein (fish, poultry, beef) should consist of no more
  than 3 to 5 oz. per meal.
• Eggs should be 5 whites or 2 whole eggs.
• Plant protein portions should be 1/2 cup for legumes
  and about 1 to 2 oz. for nuts and seeds.
• Carbs like rice, oats, and other whole grains should be
  no more than 1 cup.
• Fruit and veggies are great in all amounts and colors—
  the more fruit and veggies, the better.
• Fat will fall into place (added fat—like olive oil, salad
  dressing, and others should be no more than 2 Tbsp. at
  a time).

Notes For Factor #2:

Factor #3: Quality and Purity of Calories (Quiz #10-30)

#14   Junk Food

Junk foods should be eliminated from your diet (that includes fast food, candy, pizza, ice cream, potato chips, cookies, candy, donuts, etc.)

- Desserts should be consumed sparingly, if at all.
- Fruit and yogurt are excellent alternatives, or you can consult the Diva Smart Diet Cheat Sheet for other options.

EVEN IF YOU'RE YOUNG, LIKE JUNKSTER, JUNK FOOD NEGATIVELY AFFECTS YOUR GROWING BODY, AND CONSUMING TOO MUCH WILL EVENTUALLY CAUSE OBESITY AND POOR HEALTH!

JUNKSTER

#15   Total Daily Fat Intake (grams)

Keep your fat consumption to no more than 30 grams per day. (This also applies to "good" fats too).

#16   Total Daily Sugar Intake (grams)

Avoid table sugar, and steer clear of products with high fructose corn syrup and other sugar derivatives.

- Added sugars should equal no more than 50 grams per day, though less is preferable.
- Four extra sweeteners allowed: honey, agave nectar, natural fruit spreads, and applesauce (consumed sparingly).

#17   Sugar Substitutes (artificial sweeteners)

Avoid currently available artificial sweeteners. And pay attention when new products are introduced into the market.

SHOOG EATS SO MANY FOODS THAT ARE HIGH IN SUGAR, SUGAR DERIVATIVES, AND ARTIFICIAL SWEETENERS THAT SHE HAS BECOME FLABBY, UNHEALTHY, AND ADDICTED TO THESE ITEMS. DON'T LET THIS HAPPEN TO YOU!

#18   Total Daily Sodium Intake (milligrams)

Keep your daily sodium-to-calorie ratio at approximately 1 milligram per calorie (or less), balancing sodium with other minerals.

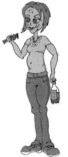

SHOOG

- Since sodium exists in food naturally, you will not need to salt your food.
- Don't use table salt, and try to eliminate salt and high-sodium products when cooking.
- Simply reducing the amount of highly processed, packaged, and man-made foods you consume will eliminate a great deal of sodium from your diet.
- Dining out is also a major factor in a high-sodium diet, so be cautious when eating at restaurants.

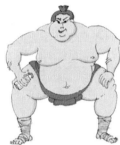

MONITORING YOUR SODIUM INTAKE REDUCES WATER RETENTION AND STRAIN ON YOUR CARDIOVASCULAR SYSTEM AND KIDNEYS—SO YOU WON'T END UP LOOKING AND FEELING LIKE SODI SUMO—BLOATED AND STIFF!

SODI SUMO

For a complete list of quality foods see Diva Reduction Good Food Choices At-a-Glance—PART SIX (pages 229-253).

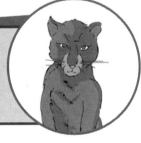

#19   Quality Protein Intake

Total daily protein should be around 100-120 grams per day (less if you ar not active).

✻Animal protein—choose from the following:
- Wild, fresh-water fish with fins and scales
- Avoid certain seafood, like shrimp, scallops, and swordfish
- Kosher, organic, free-range, and grass-fed meats
  - Lean cuts of poultry (white meat without skin)
  - Lean cuts of beef (trim excess fat, and only eat beef once per month
- Eggs from organic, free-range, vegetarian hens (eat more egg whites, and egg yolks only occasionally)
- Avoid pork and limit lamb, veal, and duck

✻Processed meats and meat products are discouraged. However, freshly sliced deli meat (turkey or chicken breast) from a reputable producer is acceptable.

✱Avoid highly processed, high-sodium, and high-fat meat products, like hot dogs (and veggie dogs), bologna, ham, pastrami, and roast beef. Sausage, bacon, and dried meats like jerky or smoked salmon should also be avoided.

✱Plant protein sources are encouraged, including legumes, nuts, and seeds. Keep in mind that although the fat naturally found in nuts and seeds is "good" fat, consumption should be kept proportionally minimal. There are seven acceptable plant protein products (as long as they are high quality): soymilk, soy yogurt, soy butter, soy cheese, tofu, hummus, and nut butters.

#20   Quality Carbohydrate Intake
Total daily carbohydrate intake should be approximately 130 to 150 grams per day (more if you are active).
- Your best carbohydrate choices include unrefined whole grains (like millet, oats, quinoa, spelt) and some whole-grain products.
- At this stage, stay clear of wheat and choose gluten-free products.
- Fresh, organic vegetables and fruits in a variety of colors provide the best type of carbohydrates, so eat those in large amounts.
- Four dried fruits are approved for now: figs, raisins, dates, and prunes.

#21   Quality Fat Intake
Total daily fat intake should be around 25 to 30 grams per day (less if you want to be an Extra-Lean Diva).
- Choose "good" fats found in salmon and other fish, nuts and seeds, olives and olive oil, and other unrefined oils.
- Medium-grade fats should be kept to a minimum, including cholesterol and saturated fat-laden foods such as meat, dairy, eggs, some seafood and coconut and palm oils.
- Avoid the "bad" fats like trans fats and hydrogenated oils found in man-made products, fast food, and fried foods.

IF YOU DON'T LIMIT THE AMOUNT AND WATCH THE QUALITY OF THE FAT YOU CONSUME, YOU MAY END UP JUST LIKE SAT FAT, DRIPPING WITH FAT INSIDE AND OUT, WITH CHOLESTEROL OOZING FROM YOUR PORES!

SAT FAT

#22   Total Daily Dairy Intake

Dairy and dairy product consumption should be limited to once or twice per day, in small portions (less is better).

- Always choose organic dairy products that come from free-range and grass-fed cows! Eleven dairy products are okay to eat: milk, cottage cheese, plain yogurt, cream cheese, sour cream, real butter, skim cheese, string cheese, Parmesan, Romano, and feta cheese (make sure your selections are non- or low-fat products whenever possible).
- You can substitute with soy- or rice-based products.
- Be aware that many packaged products contain dairy-based ingredients when you are factoring dairy intake into your diet.

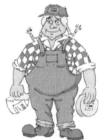

IF YOUR DAIRY INTAKE IS TOO HIGH (ESPECIALLY NON-ORGANIC) YOU MAY END UP CONSUMING MANY UNWANTED HORMONES, LIKE THE DAIRY MAIDEN.

DAIRY MAIDEN

#23   Clean Calories

Become a label reader—only buy products with five ingredients or less, unless you're well aware of their quality.

- This includes all packaged, canned, or frozen foods, and man-made food products.
- It is also important to look for ingredients that may clash with your personal dietary requirements (especially regarding medical conditions like diabetes, gluten sensitivity, lactose intolerance, etc.).

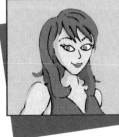

"Stick with the core of MY DIVA DIET and you will reap the rewards of a better body, better health, and a better attitude. You will also become a part of the effort toward improving our environment and discouraging mass production of animals for food, helping to alleviate animal cruelty."

338

Paw Food Guide

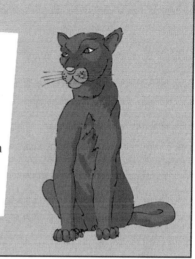

- Clean and pure foods—natural, fresh, organic, and kosher
- Lean, healthy, fibrous, and *alive* foods
- Foods made by nature for human consumption
- Carefully chosen man-made or man-manipulated foods

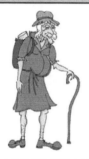

TRANNY GRANNY

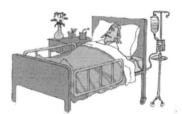

MRS. REGRET

#24   Purity of Calories

EATING CLEAN, PURE CALORIES WILL ENSURE YOU DON'T END UP LIKE TRANNY GRANNY (SHE'S ONLY 42!)—UNHEALTHY, AGING TOO FAST, AND UNABLE TO FUNCTION. MRS. REGRET ALSO FELL VICTIM TO AN UNKNOWN CULPRIT—HER BODY IS WEAK AND SUFFERING FROM A MYSTERIOUS ILLNESS. SHE WOULD BE SO MUCH HEALTHIER IF SHE HAD PAID MORE ATTENTION TO THE QUALITY OF THE FOODS SHE CONSUMED!

#25   White Flour Intake

Stay away from white flour. It is highly processed, and all nutrients have been leached away.

- The Diva Reduction Phase is a flourless diet plan, so avoid bread and pasta for now. Flour made products may be added in Phase Two—Diva Maintenance—make sure to consume only whole-grain, high-protein, high-fiber bread and pasta without too many preservatives or additives.

- Avoid other flour-based products like pancakes, waffles, muffins, and tortillas. Later in the program you can integrate these items as long as the flour used is not highly processed and the other ingredients are pure.
- There are seven grain products to choose from: rice milk, rice cakes, corn thins, spelt cakes, sprouted corn tortillas, mochi, and some cereals. See the Diva Reduction Safe Cereal List—PART SIX (pages 254-255)

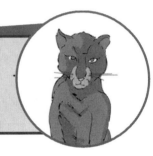

"Whole grains and grain products should never outweigh your consumption of fresh fruits and vegetables." Always ask, "Where's the fiber"?

IF YOUR DIET CONTAINS TOO MUCH WHITE FLOUR, YOU WILL END UP FAT, BLOATED, CONSTIPATED, AND PUZZLED—JUST LIKE MR. BAKERMAN!

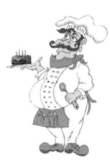

#26   Total Daily Fiber Intake (grams)
Eat approximately 25-35 grams of fiber each day. Make sure you eat fresh vegetables, fruits, whole grains, legumes, nuts, and seeds every day, while avoiding processed and man-made foods.

MR. BAKERMAN

#27   Food, Sports, Energy, and Protein Bars
        These should be avoided during Phase One—Diva Reduction but they may be used as an emergency snack if they have high-quality ingredients.

#28   Sauces, Salad Dressing, and Condiment Intake
        Keep your condiment intake to a minimum. This also includes dressings, sauces, dips and spreads. Ingredients should be examined thoroughly and the products should be used moderately.

#29   Cooking and Seasoning: Fruits, Vegetables, Herbs, and Spices
        Always monitor how your food is prepared. See our Food Prep/Cooking Guide—PART FIVE (pages 206-215), MY DIVA DIET Restaurant Eating Guide—PART SIX (pages 268-276), and Herbs and Spice—PART SEVEN (pages 299-304).

#30 Supplement Intake: (Vitamins, Minerals, and Others)
Supplements should never be used to replace your diet, only to enhance it.
Remember, there is no "miracle pill" that will make you healthy & fit or
add years to your life, and that includes pills labeled "natural".

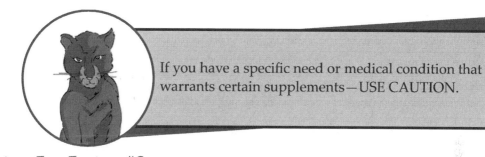

If you have a specific need or medical condition that
warrants certain supplements—USE CAUTION.

Notes For Factor #3:

Factor #4: Restrictive and Unbalanced Dieting

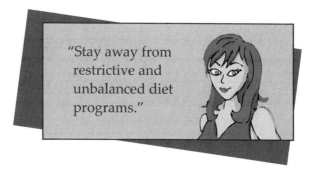

"Stay away from
restrictive and
unbalanced diet
programs."

#31 Restrictive and Unbalanced Dieting
- No starvation
- No diet pills
- No gimmicks
- No unbalanced dieting

DON'T BELIEVE DR. PILL OR NURSE GIMMICK! DR. PILL MAY LOOK INNOCENT, BUT HE IS A SNAKE IN DISGUISE. AND NURSE GIMMICK IS SICK, MOODY, CONFUSED, AND UNABLE TO FUNCTION DUE TO ALL THE BAD DIETS SHE'S TRIED! WHY FOLLOW HER LEAD?

Notes For Factor #4:

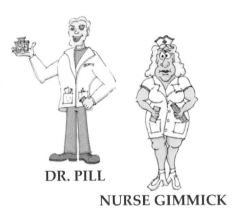

DR. PILL

NURSE GIMMICK

Factor #5: Exercise
#32   Weekly Exercise Program

Add a complete and balanced exercise program to your weekly schedule.

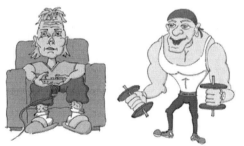

Diva 6 Components to an Effective Exercise Program
- Cardiovascular conditioning
- Strength and endurance training
- Flexibility training
- Core and balance training
- Corrective exercises
- Functional training

DON'T LET LAZINESS GET THE BEST OF YOU LIKE VEGG! THE OTHER EXTREME, THOUGH, IS JUST AS BAD! TRY TO CREATE A BALANCED, DRUG-FREE EXERCISE PROGRAM SO YOU DON'T END UP LIKE GEORGE – OUT OF BALANCE PHYSICALLY, EMOTIONALLY, AND MENTALLY, WITH MANY HEALTH PROBLEMS LURKING BENEATH THE SURFACE!

VEGG   **GEORGE GOTTA GO**

Notes For Factor #5:

MY DIVA DIET Society Guide

Diva Housewife:

It is never too early or too late to convince your kids and your spouse to adopt a healthy & fit lifestyle. You'll not only be doing them a favor, but you'll be doing yourself one as well! The best thing you can do for your children is to create good habits early.

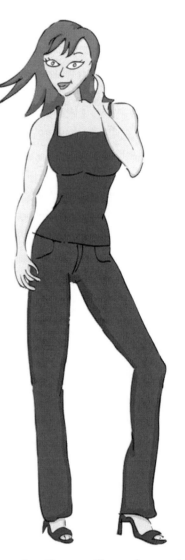

Diet:

1. Cook your healthy & fit meals and don't worry if they don't like them initially. Give them some time and explain the benefits, and their tastes buds (and attitudes) will adjust. When they get older they will thank you.

2. When you cook, make the main dish for everyone (healthy & fit), but provide a side dish of something you may not be able to eat so they don't feel deprived.
    *   Instead of a corn tortilla, they can have a flour tortilla.
    *   Even if you can't have grains late at night, it's okay if they do.
    *   Let them have a little pasta on the side, even if it is not gluten-free.
    *   Let them have a little bread when you can't. Bread dipped in olive oil and Balsamic vinegar tastes great and provides additional nutrients.

3. Plan ahead. Since you are probably busy with your family, you'll need an extra edge to make sure you stay on track with your own weight-loss program.

4. When you spend time with your friends, show them how you can have your bread, pasta, and potato too!

5. Make new friends that share your goal of living a healthy & fit lifestyle.

Exercise:

1. Make time to exercise. Maybe you can get up a half-hour before the rest of your household for a quick workout. Your exercise routine doesn't have to be a three-hour ordeal.

2. Fit in small exercises where you can. Try doing some squats while you fold laundry, or do some abdominal crunches while you catch up on your favorite TV or radio program.

3. Don't let that treadmill or those dumbbells collect dust–you can do a quick half-hour workout while you help your children with their homework.

4. Ask your spouse this question: "Honey, don't you want me to look better and be happier?" When your spouse responds 'yes', you can respond, "Well, will you help me carve out just one hour a day so I can work out and plan healthy meals for you and our family?"

Diva Single Mom:

You have the very difficult job of balancing your kids and job while incorporating a new lifestyle of exercise and proper diet. A good support system is helpful, so try to get your friends and family on board with you. While eating right and exercising may cost you a little extra time, it also means less time spent ill, with fewer trips to and less money wasted at the doctor's office. And better yet, getting in shape will give you the endurance you need to fulfill your responsibilities.

Diet:

1. Meals don't have to be expensive to be healthy. Fresh, wholesome foods aren't much more expensive, even if they're organic and kosher. It's more expensive to get takeout or eat at restaurants, and highly-processed foods often cost just as much.

2. Meals don't have to take three hours to cook. In fact, well-balanced, healthy meals are often quicker and easier to prepare. For example, cooking a yam, washing an apple and eating it with some string-cheese, cooking some wild rice in your rice cooker, or even baking some chicken while chopping veggies for a salad takes less time than preparing a fattening gourmet meal.

3. Plan ahead. Use your 3-Week Diva Diet and Exercise Calendar or your MY DIVA DIET Journal to plan meals for the week ahead.

Exercise:

1. Exercise equipment does not have to cost a fortune. Take advantage of some inexpensive home exercise equipment that can be very effective and efficient. A Swiss ball, a foam roller, dumbbells, and exercise bands cost less than $100 and provide you with all the tools you need for a workout routine that will get you more fit!

2. Exercise doesn't have to take all day. You can complete a successful workout at home in thirty minutes.

3. Depending on the ages of your kids, find ways to get outside and do some cardio:

    • If they are in a stroller—buckle them up and go.
    • If they are older—take them for a bike ride.
    • If they are "too cool" for a bike—they can skateboard while you power walk.
    • If they are teenagers—invite them to work out with you—this can create a great bonding opportunity!

4. Find other single moms in your area and buddy up with them.

5. Play a team sport—join the community softball or soccer team.

6. If you're spiritual, invite women from your place of worship to form a walking group. Since you're already used to multi-tasking, you can use your skills to advance your physical and spiritual condition at the same time!

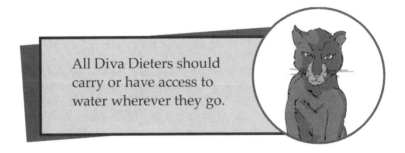

All Diva Dieters should carry or have access to water wherever they go.

Diva Career Woman:

First and foremost, good health & fitness will only help you progress in your career! It is vital to balance your personal fitness and health with the pace of your profession. As busy and important as you are, your time is limited, so try to plan your workout and diet schedule in advance. You use so many of your talents in your occupation—try to apply them to your goals of becoming leaner, stronger, and more vivacious, and to creating longevity not only in your career but in your life as well.

Diet:

1. When preparing a meal, make a little extra for the next day at work. Soups and salads are great for that.

2. Purchase a cooler and stock it with healthy foods for the day, so you're not tempted to eat the birthday cake, cookies, brownies, and leftover spinach dip your coworkers leave sitting on the break-room table at work.

3. Carry the MY DIVA DIET Restaurant Eating Guide in your bag for the times you go out to lunch with a colleague.

4. Set an alarm (cell phones work great for this!) to remind you to eat every three to four hours.

5. At happy hour, drink your water in a cocktail or wine glass. You'll be part of the party, but you won't have to deal with all the additional calories (or tomorrow morning's hangover)!

Exercise:

1. If you can join a gym, do it. Once you're acquainted with the facilities, find yourself a workout buddy.

2. Try to exercise before work if you think you may be too tired at the end of the day. If mornings don't work, try to exercise during lunch.

3. If a gym just isn't your thing, you can always rely on your home workout gear and personalized program.

4. Exercise does not have to be an all-or-nothing situation. Exercising for only thirty minutes two times per week constitutes a beneficial workout routine–something is better than nothing!

5. There are simple things you can do to be more physically active.
   - While sitting at the computer, try some isometric contractions (squeeze specific muscle groups like your abdominals or glutes)
   - Instead of riding the elevator, take the stairs.
   - Park further away from your work building. The extra walking will add up.
   - If you have pets, take them for long walks on your days off. They'll love it, and it will be good for you!

Diva College Girl & Diva Career Girl:

For the younger generation of females, keep in mind that what you do today impacts your tomorrow and this holds true when it comes to your decisions on diet and exercise. If you are in college or already working, you can set an example for your friends and family by cooking and eating right and exercising regularly. You can show them how cool and fun it is to look "smokin' hot" and rarely get sick!

Diet:

1. Don't worry about what kind of food you were raised with. It's your body, and now that you're an adult it's your responsibility to take care of it.

2. Set your alarm to wake you up at least ten minutes earlier in the morning so you can fit in a balanced breakfast.

3. Carry your MY DIVA DIET Restaurant Eating Guide in your purse (or backpack) for a handy reference everywhere you go.

4. Keep the Paw Fast Food Five Guide readily available for those times you need a quick on-the-go meal idea.

5. Try to pack your own meals for an entire day, so you can eat healthy while on campus or at work.

6. Purchase a small cooler and keep it in your car so you can enjoy cold lunches and snacks at school and at work.

7. Plan and write out your daily meals and shop weekly. If you're on a tight budget, weekly shopping will help you avoid wasting food and money.

8. Regularly volunteer to be the designated driver. It's a great way to avoid extra calories, and everybody's safer because of you!

Exercise:

1. If you can afford it, hire a fitness trainer to get you started. Your trainer can motivate you and turn you into a lean, sexy machine.

2. Find a gym buddy.

3. Park your car somewhere on or off-campus or further from your place of employment where you have to walk a bit further than usual.

4. If you live close to work or school, you could walk or ride your bike.

Diva Teen:

If you are in high school (or middle school), you can show your friends and even your parents the best way to diet. You can teach them how to get healthy & fit in a safe and lasting way. You just may be the generation that reverses your family's "diet curse" and ends up with a fit and fabulous figure forever!

Diet:

1. Eat a healthy breakfast. Try a yam—it's a great source for hours of energy.
2. Skip the dreadful school lunch program—it never tastes like food anyway.
3. You're old enough to pack your own lunch—or at least to decide what you want.
4. Make sure you pack some healthy snacks for your long day at school: baby carrots and low-fat ranch dressing, an apple and string cheese, or banana and nut butter.
5. Get involved in meal planning with your parents. It's time to voice your opinion and make your own good choices.
6. Make a grocery list for your parents and use the MY DIVA DIET Grocery Shopping Guide as well as the Diva Reduction Good Food Choices At-a-Glance section.
7. Try to find a new, healthy recipe so you and your family can have fun making it into a Diva Reduction Recipe (this may be the time to learn how to cook).
8. Don't let your parents buy you junk food. Just say "no" and help them find something better.

Exercise:

1. Get involved in a sports program or sports team. Who knows, maybe it will lead to bigger things and you'll grace magazine covers as the next tennis, golf, basketball, track, volleyball, or karate star!
2. Create your own workout group with some friends and stick to it two to three times a week.
3. Enlist your family in a weekend activity, like a tennis match or basketball game.

Diva Handicapped/ Disabled Woman:

Of all people, you know how important it is to maintain good health & fitness levels. Your body, regardless of your disability, will perform at its highest level of function when your diet and exercise regimen is on-target. You'll reap rewards in small increments of happiness, healing, and strength.

Support systems are key, so find friends, family, local church groups and others who are in situations similar to yours and motivate one another toward health & fitness.

Diet:

1. Do some research on your particular disability and learn how diet can facilitate your goals (whether you are trying to lose fat or gain lean body mass) and your healing. It will be informative and can also serve as a great motivator.

2. Whether or not you're on a tight budget, write out a weekly meal plan and stick to it. This will keep you on track, save you money, and keep you from wasting food.

3. Prepare foods in their natural form: they taste better, are better for you, and will save you time when cooking.

4. If you have an eventful day planned, you should pack a cooler with fresh snacks like fruits, veggies, nuts, and water.

Exercise:

1. If you can, hire a Physical Therapist or qualified Fitness Professional to design an exercise program for you. The cost is minimal compared to the benefits it will provide.

2. When watching TV or a movie, try to stretch all the body parts you can; just move your body around as much as possible. It feels great and promotes blood flow.

3. Grab a friend and engage in physical activity as often as possible.

4. Get outdoors: it's a natural motivator–you'll be happier and more healthful!

Diva Retired Woman:

With all the time you have, you should be fit as a fiddle! It's never too late to start. You can get into good shape, increase your energy level, improve your posture, feel better, and even relieve some of the ailments you may have been suffering for years.

Diet:

1. Plan and write out your daily meals, stick to your plan, and shop accordingly.

2. Take a cooking class with your spouse or friends, or create your own "Cook a Fit Recipe Night".

3. Experiment with wholesome foods. A little change may be fun—stir the pot, so to speak! For example: try quinoa instead of oatmeal for breakfast.

4. Make a large amount of soup, then freeze it for a quick lunch or dinner another day.

Exercise:

1. If you don't have dog, walk your spouse! Getting outdoors is energizing and healthy.

2. If your activity level has been low, start slowly by taking short walks (even on a treadmill). You can increase your walking time and pace when you feel ready.

3. If you have joint pain, you can try swimming or exercises done in a pool. The water relieves pressure on your joints (so you can exercise pain-free) and creates added resistance, which is great for building strength and muscle mass.

4. Try listening to an iPod when you walk. You will be amazed how the time flies by when you are listening to your favorite music (whether it's Elvis or Beethoven).

5. Maintain your flexibility by adding a ten-minute stretching session to your routine before you go to bed, or right after your early morning walk.

6. Enlist a friend and switch off doing your favorite activities, or try something new, like golf, swimming, yoga, or aerobics classes.

7. Keep an open mind about weight training. It really does constitute a large part of "the fountain of youth" by maintaining healthy, well-developed muscles.

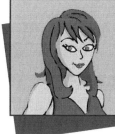

"If *we* spent more time exercising and eating right we would spend less time being sick, less money on medications, less time and money at the doctor's office and the beauty parlor, and even less money on clothes and make-up, because we would feel so much better about ourselves."

Diva Worksheet #2
Diva Diet Quiz Summary—
The Five Factors Scores and Diet Villains Exposed

Diva Diet Quiz Score = _____

MY Diet Grade—put your grade here = _____

How can I improve my overall diet and exercise program?
Write notes based on your grades and where you think you can improve.

The Five Factors Affecting Body Fat and Health Scores

Transfer your factor totals from the Diva Diet Quiz (PART THREE) to this worksheet. Circle the score you received and see how you fare for each of the Five Factors, while exposing your personal Diet Villains. Make notes on how you can fix a factor and defeat your personal Diet Villains (for a full explanation of the Five Factors and Diet Villains, see PART TWO).

Factor #1   Liquid Consumption

Great	Good	Needs Improvement	Poor
170 to 101	**100 to 0**	**-1 to -100**	**-101 to -190**

Defeat Your Diet Villains!

POPS   **CAFF**   **AL AND COLE**

Notes:

Factor #2   Quantity & Distribution of Daily Calories

Great	Good	Needs Improvement	Poor
110 to 51	**50 to 0**	**-1 to -65**	**-66 to -125**

Notes:

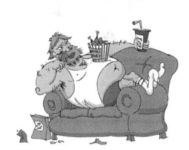

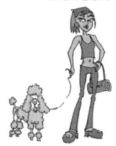

Defeat Your Diet Villains!

**GIRLIE DIE AND
HER POODLE, IT**

JOE STUFFT

Factor #3   Quality & Purity of Calories

Great	Good	Needs Improvement	Poor
435 to 221	**220 to 0**	**-1 to -220**	**-221 to -435**

JUNKSTER   **SHOOG**   **SODI SUMO**   **SAT FAT**

Defeat Your Diet Villains!

DAIRY MAIDEN **TRANNY GRANNY**   **MRS. REGRET**   **MR. BAKERMAN**

Notes:

Factor #4   Restrictive & Unbalanced Dieting

Great	Good	Needs Improvement	Poor
50 to 41	**40 to 0**	**-1 to -40**	**-41 to -50**

Notes:

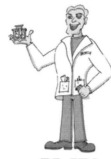 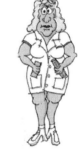

DR. PILL   **NURSE GIMMICK**

Defeat Your Diet Villains!

Factor #5   Exercise

Great	Good	Needs Improvement	Poor
65 to 31	**30 to 0**	**-1 to -30**	**-31 to -65**

Notes:

Defeat Your Diet Villains!

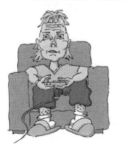 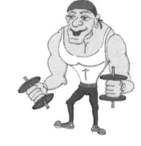

VEGG   **GEORGE GOTTA GO**

Diva Worksheet #3
3-Day Diet Analysis Instructions & Food Diary Sheets

Step 1
Find a food dictionary that lists calories, grams of protein, carbohydrates, and fats. It's also a good idea to count grams of fiber, milligrams of sodium, and grams of sugar. We recommend The Corinne Netzer Encyclopedia of Food Values, Prevention Magazine's Nutrition Advisor and The World's Healthiest Foods, by George Mateljan. There are also many other books and websites that can help you find the nutritional value of different foods and ingredients. You can find food values online at www.calorieking.com and www.fitday.com.

Step 2
Use the food diary sheets provided and note the date first. Then, within the appropriate meal number, write down the time of meal, name of food item and the amount consumed (use your best estimate).

Step 3
Use your food dictionary or website to fill in the other information for each meal. Calories, grams of protein, carbohydrates, fat, and fiber should be listed. Sodium is measured in milligrams.

Step 4
Total the numbers for each meal in to the "total meal" section, this will help you with portion control. At the end of each day, total all the meals you have eaten to get a record of your daily calories, protein (grams), carbohydrates (grams), fat (grams), fiber (grams), and sodium (milligrams).

Step 5
Repeat Steps 2-4 for at least three days, but seven days is ideal because our eating habits tend to vary on weekends.

Step 6
If you want to take the process further, you can transfer your totals to Diva Worksheet #4 (found in the following pages 363 to 365) in order to:
- Calculate your daily nutrient ratio using the Paw Guide to Calculating Your Nutrient Ratio
- Compare your daily nutrient ratio to the Paw Daily Nutrient Ratio Guide
- Compare your nutrients in grams to the Paw Daily Nutrient Guide

Food Diary Sheets

MY Food Diary Worksheet: Day 1							
Name:							
Day:			Date:				

Meal #1
Time:

Food Item	Amount	Calories	Protein/g	Carbs/g	Fat/g	Fiber/g	Sodium/mg
Total Meal #1:							

Notes:

Meal #2
Time:

Food Item	Amount	Calories	Protein/g	Carbs/g	Fat/g	Fiber/g	Sodium/mg
Total Meal #2:							

Notes:

Meal #3 Time:							
Food Item	Amount	Calories	Protein/g	Carbs/g	Fat/g	Fiber/g	Sodium/mg
Total Meal #3:							
Notes:							

Meal #4 Time:							
Food Item	Amount	Calories	Protein/g	Carbs/g	Fat/g	Fiber/g	Sodium/mg
Total Meal #4:							
Notes:							

Total Day 1 Calories:	
Protein (grams):	
Carbohydrates (grams):	
Fat (grams):	
Fiber (grams):	
Sodium (milligrams):	

MY Food Diary Worksheet: Day 2

Name:

Day:	Date:

Meal #1
Time:

Food Item	Amount	Calories	Protein/g	Carbs/g	Fat/g	Fiber/g	Sodium/mg
Total Meal #1:							
Notes:							

Meal #2
Time:

Food Item	Amount	Calories	Protein/g	Carbs/g	Fat/g	Fiber/g	Sodium/mg
Total Meal #2:							
Notes:							

Meal #3 Time:							
Food Item	Amount	Calories	Protein/g	Carbs/g	Fat/g	Fiber/g	Sodium/mg
Total Meal #3:							
Notes:							

Meal #4 Time:							
Food Item	Amount	Calories	Protein/g	Carbs/g	Fat/g	Fiber/g	Sodium/mg
Total Meal #4:							
Notes:							

Total Day 2 Calories:	
Protein (grams):	
Carbohydrates (grams):	
Fat (grams):	
Fiber (grams):	
Sodium (milligrams):	

MY Food Diary Worksheet: Day 3

Name:							
Day:			Date:				

Meal #1
Time:

Food Item	Amount	Calories	Protein/g	Carbs/g	Fat/g	Fiber/g	Sodium/mg
Total Meal #1:							

Notes:

Meal #2
Time:

Food Item	Amount	Calories	Protein/g	Carbs/g	Fat/g	Fiber/g	Sodium/mg
Total Meal #2:							

Notes:

Meal #3 Time:							
Food Item	Amount	Calories	Protein/g	Carbs/g	Fat/g	Fiber/g	Sodium/mg
Total Meal #3:							
Notes:							

Meal #4 Time:							
Food Item	Amount	Calories	Protein/g	Carbs/g	Fat/g	Fiber/g	Sodium/mg
Total Meal #4:							
Notes:							

Total Day 3 Calories:	
Protein (grams):	
Carbohydrates (grams):	
Fat (grams):	
Fiber (grams):	
Sodium (milligrams):	

Diva Worksheet #4
3-Day Diet Analysis Totals:
Daily Calories and Nutrient Totals—Nutrient Ratio Calculations

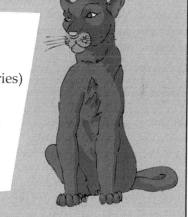

Paw Guide to Calculating
Your Nutrient Ratio

- (Total protein grams x 4) divided by (total calories)
  = **% protein**
- (Total carb grams x 4) divided by (total calories)
  = **% carbs**
- (Total fat grams x 9) divided by (total calories)
  = **% fat**

MY Daily Calories and Nutrient Totals						
Day 1	Calories	Protein (g)	Carbs (g)	Fat (g)	Fiber (g)	Sodium (mg)
Day 2	Calories	Protein (g)	Carbs (g)	Fat (g)	Fiber (g)	Sodium (mg)
Day 3	Calories	Protein (g)	Carbs (g)	Fat (g)	Fiber (g)	Sodium (mg)

MY Daily Nutrient Ratio*	Day One		
Total Protein (g)	x4 =	/Total Calories =	% protein
Total Carbs (g)	x4 =	/Total Calories =	% carbs
Total Fat (g)	x9 =	/Total Calories =	% fat

MY Daily Nutrient Ratio*	Day Two		
Total Protein (g)	x4 =	/Total Calories =	% protein
Total Carbs (g)	x4 =	/Total Calories =	% carbs
Total Fat (g)	x9 =	/Total Calories =	% fat

MY Daily Nutrient Ratio*	Day Three		
Total Protein (g)	x4 =	/Total Calories =	% protein
Total Carbs (g)	x4 =	/Total Calories =	% carbs
Total Fat (g)	x9 =	/Total Calories =	% fat
*Compare your totals to the following Paw Guides			

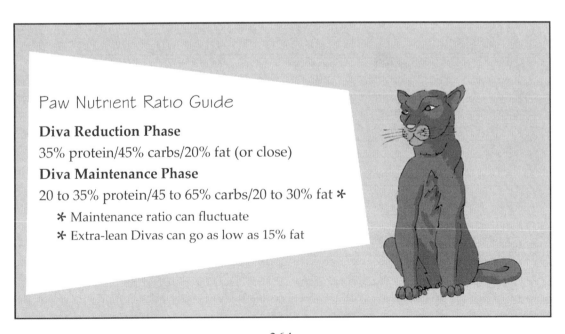

Paw Nutrient Ratio Guide

Diva Reduction Phase
35% protein/45% carbs/20% fat (or close)
Diva Maintenance Phase
20 to 35% protein/45 to 65% carbs/20 to 30% fat ✶
   ✶ Maintenance ratio can fluctuate
   ✶ Extra-lean Divas can go as low as 15% fat

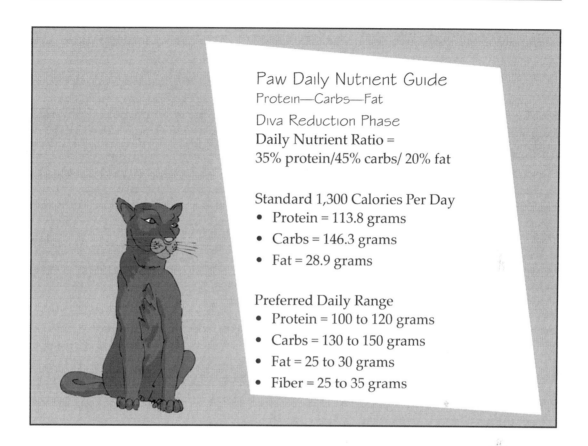

Paw Daily Nutrient Guide
Protein—Carbs—Fat

Diva Reduction Phase
Daily Nutrient Ratio =
35% protein/45% carbs/ 20% fat

Standard 1,300 Calories Per Day
- Protein = 113.8 grams
- Carbs = 146.3 grams
- Fat = 28.9 grams

Preferred Daily Range
- Protein = 100 to 120 grams
- Carbs = 130 to 150 grams
- Fat = 25 to 30 grams
- Fiber = 25 to 35 grams

Diva Worksheet #5
Personal Goals:
Instructions & MY DIVA DIET Goal Sheet

The goal of MY DIVA DIET is very simple: Lose Fat—Gain Health! Look, feel, and function better—and live longer!

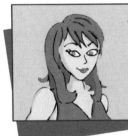

"To decrease body fat (including cellulite) while increasing health; to get lean, fit and BE a better woman—these are the goals of all Diva Dieters. We hope that all women are successful in this endeavor, as well as all other noble and pure adventures."

Ms. Diva may have outlined the general goal for your MY DIVA DIET program, but in order to succeed you need to be more specific and establish your own personal goals. As women, our bodies vary greatly in weight, body-fat level, structure, and size. We also have individual lifestyles, motivations, and overall goals that require personalized attention. We recognize this, so go ahead and make this your place to set personal goals. The key is to set realistic goals, so that you can be sure to succeed!

When you're ready to set your goals, the first step is to test your body fat. Your local fitness center is an excellent resource, or you can contact a Certified Personal Trainer or even your physician.

The second step is to get accurate measurements. A great way to monitor your progress is by keeping track of your measurements. Have a friend or Certified Personal Trainer help you, and you may even want to track your clothing size throughout your program. Record your numbers in Diva Worksheet #5 as well as at the beginning of your Progress Report—Diva Worksheet #6.

Note on Health:
Consider a visit to your physician to get a physical examination. If you want to track your cholesterol, blood pressure, heart rate, bone density, or other medical concerns, your physician will be able to help you. Make a note of any medications you may be taking, including over-the-counter drugs. It's possible that you'll be able to eliminate

the need for some of those pills by improving your overall health & fitness levels through proper eating and exercise!

Body Composition and Goals

It is important that you understand why obtaining your body composition is so critical —especially when you're trying to reduce body fat.

- First, body composition is a true gauge of the components that make up your body weight, whether you are 100 or 200 pounds.
- Second, when you begin to exercise, your weight may not fluctuate at all—this is due to a possible increase in muscle mass.
- Third, the information you discover can help you make peace with your body weight, as well as provide you with a more relevant tool for monitoring your progress.

The MY DIVA DIET goal for body fat is 17-25%.

This range means that your body-fat levels are excellent to acceptable, even at 22% body fat you are in good shape while at 25% your body fat will be much lower than the majority of the population. It is also possible for athletic Divas and extra-lean Divas to consider the 12-16% body-fat range.

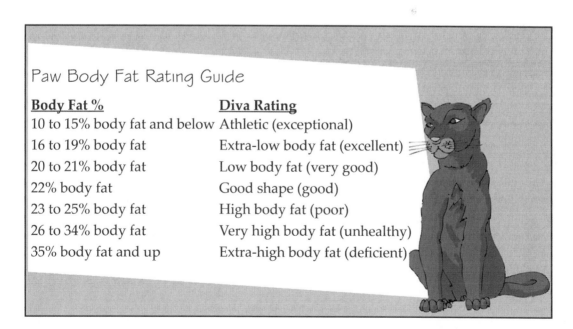

Paw Body Fat Rating Guide

Body Fat %	Diva Rating
10 to 15% body fat and below	Athletic (exceptional)
16 to 19% body fat	Extra-low body fat (excellent)
20 to 21% body fat	Low body fat (very good)
22% body fat	Good shape (good)
23 to 25% body fat	High body fat (poor)
26 to 34% body fat	Very high body fat (unhealthy)
35% body fat and up	Extra-high body fat (deficient)

However, if you have an initial body-fat level in the 30s, or even 40-50%, don't despair! Start yourself off with a short-term goal. After you've accomplished that goal, re-evaluate and set another goal. Repeat this process until you've reached your long-term goals. Then you can move on to a maintenance plan.

Keep in mind that everyone is different, and if you are happy at the 20% level, stay there. Not all Diva Dieters need to go for the ultimate in low body fat but understand that it is an attainable goal for those who want it. MY DIVA DIET is for women of all shapes and sizes who want to work toward becoming leaner and healthier.

Another point to consider is that we never want to be locked into a number. Try to create a range, not only for your body-fat percentage but for your weight as well. This allows for the occasional special circumstances in life that cause us to overeat or neglect to exercise, like weddings, holidays, and even sick days, without causing us to feel like we've failed ourselves or our weight-loss program.

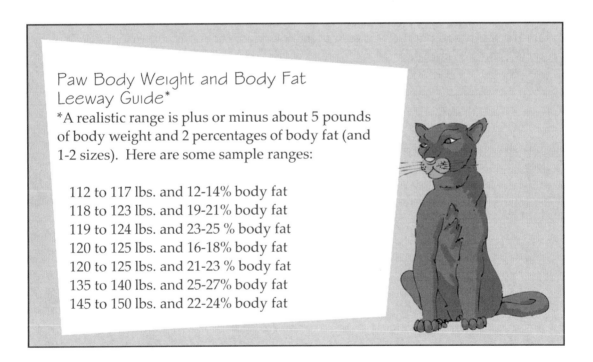

Paw Body Weight and Body Fat Leeway Guide*
*A realistic range is plus or minus about 5 pounds of body weight and 2 percentages of body fat (and 1-2 sizes). Here are some sample ranges:

112 to 117 lbs. and 12-14% body fat
118 to 123 lbs. and 19-21% body fat
119 to 124 lbs. and 23-25 % body fat
120 to 125 lbs. and 16-18% body fat
120 to 125 lbs. and 21-23 % body fat
135 to 140 lbs. and 25-27% body fat
145 to 150 lbs. and 22-24% body fat

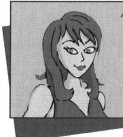

"Setting a range gives us boundaries and freedom at the same time. What a great way to live! If we go to an extreme in either direction—no boundaries or no freedom—we are more apt to fail. Our personal boundaries will also keep us from regaining too much weight ever."

MY DIVA DIET Goal Sheet

You need more than a bathroom scale to set and track your fitness goals! A skin-fold caliper and a tape measure are two important tools to which you should have access. Consider an accurate assessment of your clothing size, and don't fear a "before" photo in a swimsuit. It's a powerful tool, and you'll be amazed at how motivational it can be—especially when you lose twenty pounds of fat, gain four pounds of lean body mass, lose twelve inches in measurements, drop three dress sizes, and get daily compliments about how great you look!

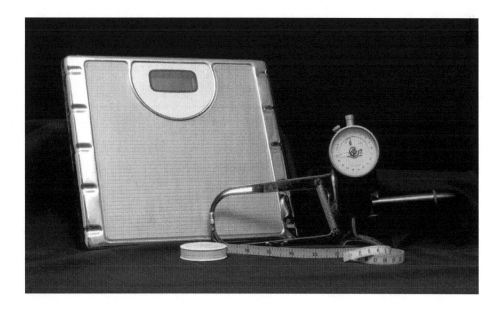

Calculate your desired weight and body-fat percentage, clothing size, and any other information you may want to track.

MY DIVA DIET Goal Sheet			
Name:			
My Range			
Weight(Lb)	From:	To:	
Fat (%)	From:	To:	
Size	From:	To:	
	Initial Numbers	Goal Numbers	
Weight (Lb):			
Body Fat (%):			
Lean Body Mass (Lb)*:			
Fat (Lb)*:			
Dress Size:			
Pant Size:			
Blouse Size:			
Fat (Lb) Loss:			
LBM Gain/Loss:			
# Weeks to Goal:			
Date of Goal:			
Notes			

*Multiply your weight in pounds by your body fat in percentage points. For example, 145 lbs x 0.27 (27% body fat) equals 39.15. This figure represents your body fat in pounds, which you subtract from your total weight to obtain your lean body mass (LBM). In this example, LBM equals 105.85 pounds.

"Be realistic, but stay motivated!"

Paw Goal-Setting Guide
(Example Scenario)

Current Status:
- You weigh 145 pounds and have 27% body fat.
  - This means that your lean body mass is 105.85 pounds and you have 39.15 pounds of fat.

Your first goal:
- You set your first goal at a weight of 132 pounds and 22% body fat.
  - This means that you would need to lose 13 pounds of body weight and 5% body fat, which would put your lean body mass at 102.96 pounds and 29.04 pounds of fat.
- Overall, your loss totals would have to equal about 10 pounds of fat and 3 pounds of lean body mass to meet this goal.

Your estimated time frame:
- To determine how long it would take for you to reach your goal, divide the required 10 pounds of fat loss by 1 or 2 pounds per week. The actual amount you lose will depend on your level of commitment to your diet and exercise regimen —the more committed you are, the more weight you will lose per week.
  - In this example, you would meet your goals in approximately 5-10 weeks!

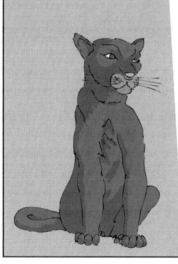

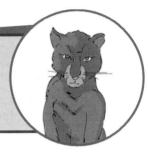

If you don't want to deal with the calculations on your own, have your body fat tested and goals set by a Fitness Professional.

Important Information About Fat Loss:

1) Realistically and safely, you can lose only one to two pounds of fat per week.

2) At the beginning of any diet program you can lose five to fifteen pounds of weight, or more, quickly. However, this initial weight loss usually consists of water weight, glycogen, and only a small percentage of fat.

3) Losing fat may take longer if:
   - You have a medical condition that would inhibit weight loss
   - You take certain medications
   - You are transitioning from a very restrictive or starvation-type of diet program
   - You choose not to exercise

4) As you continue to lose weight and body fat, the rate at which you lose slows down due to a natural protective mechanism. For example: if you have fifty pounds to lose, the first twenty pounds may be relatively easy. However, as you become lighter and leaner you have to be smarter and more aggressive to get to the next level, eventually reaching your ultimate fat loss goals.

5) Note for Extra-Lean Divas: If you're already light and lean (for example, 110 to 125 lbs and 15-18% body fat), it will be slightly more difficult to lose fat and/or weight. Don't worry though, you can still reach your goals—you just have to work smarter and be patient.

Body Composition Information

When you're serious about reducing fat, the most important thing to consider is not your total body weight but rather what makes up that weight. This is referred to as your "body composition".

Your body composition is a combination of your lean body mass (LBM) (skin, bones, hair, organs, muscle, and water) and your body fat (BF). Your own ideal weight is the weight at which your lean mass and fat mass are combined in the correct proportion for health, wellness, and aesthetics. When you are in shape, you have a proportionally higher amount of lean body weight and a lower amount of body fat, regardless of what you weigh.

Body composition analysis is an important consideration when evaluating health and risk factors, and is essential when you follow a weight-reduction program. Too much fat not only alters your appearance, but it also puts additional strain on your joints and increases your risk for other health problems. Too little fat isn't good either; it may mean your body isn't functioning at its full potential.

Traditional weight scales can't differentiate between how many pounds of lean mass or fat are on your body (percent fat). The best way to identify your percent fat and your personal correct weight is to measure your body composition. Also, if you have a specific "dream" weight, taking your body composition measurements will determine whether that goal is attainable, or whether it's an unrealistic fantasy.

FAQ
What is cellulite anyway?
We all seem to know what body fat is, and we're well aware of its presence on our own bodies, but there are some misconceptions about that "ugly" cottage cheese-like stuff that lies just under our skin, constantly embarrassing us. We seem to think it's a "special" fat; however, a little education on the subject can clear up some of the mystery behind what cellulite is and what it is not. Basically cellulite is a collection of fat that is pushed against the connective tissue beneath our skin. The uneven distribution is what causes the surface of the skin to dimple. There are many reasons why some women have more visible cellulite than others: genetics, gender, age, skin thickness, and the amount of fat you carry on your body (as well as where you carry it) are all factors. But there is nothing special about cellulite and there are no secret lotions that will get rid of it. By reducing your overall level of body fat, your cellulite will either

melt away or fade to a tolerable level. The lower your body-fat level, the less cellulite you will have.

What about the location of my fat?
Generally, women tend to carry fat on the hips, thighs, buttocks, and even around the abdominal area, while men store fat in the torso, often around the stomach. Genetics, gender, age, and ethnicity all play a role in where your body stores its fat.

What is a good body fat percentage for a woman?
The range of body fat considered healthy & fit for women is 12-22%. Research has proven that a body-fat level higher than this increases risk of coronary heart disease, diabetes, and cancer. Your attainable goal, or correct weight, should fall in that range, close to 20%. Unfortunately, the average American woman has a body fat percentage of over 33%, which is not healthy and is considered obese.

How is my age related to my body fat level?
Body composition is an age-dependent variable because as we age, there is a natural loss of muscle mass and water, with a corresponding increase in body fat. This change greatly depends on an individual's lifestyle and nutritional habits. The more physically active you are, the greater the percentage of lean body mass you will maintain, and the less fat you will develop compared to a more sedentary person—no matter what your age is!

What about water weight?
Body composition is a study of water, fat, and lean body mass. All of these factors must be considered when conducting a proper body composition analysis. A woman's body is made up of approximately 60% water. Since adipose (fat) tissue essentially contains no water, the percentage of water for an obese individual is significantly lower than that of a non-obese individual. Altering the ratio of lean tissue to fat tissue is as simple as engaging in exercise and proper nutritional habits.

What about losing weight fast?
Diets that promise incredible weight loss in a matter of days or even weeks may sound good when you're thinking about stepping on the scale, but the claims are misleading. In fact, initial weight loss is mostly water. This is because these types of diets are usually low in calories and carbohydrates, resulting in rapid water and glycogen loss. These type of diets will eventually lead to loss in muscle mass rather than fat loss, which will result in a slower metabolism.

How does exercise contribute to body fat loss?

It is well-known that exercise burns calories, but it also keeps your metabolic rate at an increased level for hours afterward. Strength training makes you look firmer and results in an increase of lean body mass, which increases your metabolic rate. Cardiovascular conditioning is great for your heart and lungs, and it burns calories and fat, though it's not as effective as strength training is in the development of lean body mass. The key to getting leaner is to incorporate both cardio and strength training into your exercise routine.

In fact, in order to reap all of the best benefits exercise has to offer—you should incorporate all of the following components to your routine:

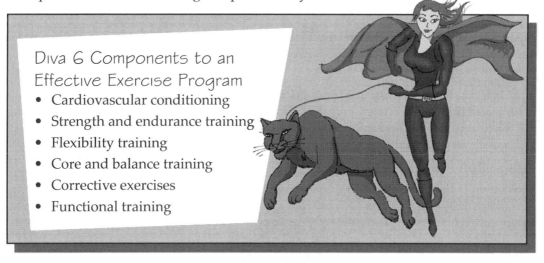

Diva 6 Components to an
Effective Exercise Program
- Cardiovascular conditioning
- Strength and endurance training
- Flexibility training
- Core and balance training
- Corrective exercises
- Functional training

Can I spot-reduce fat?

This is a common misconception. Exercise will firm the muscles under a layer of fat but it will not lead to fat reduction in a particular area. Fat storage is systematic, and its introduction to or reduction from the body is different for each person, as is the area in which each individual

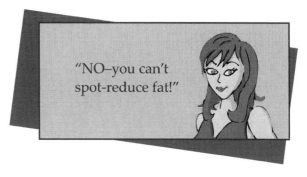

"NO–you can't spot-reduce fat!"

stores fat on her body. Because of this, two women may both have 20% body fat, but the shapes of their bodies may be completely different based on where the majority of each woman's fat is stored. This is all due to the degree of variability between individuals—it's what makes us unique.

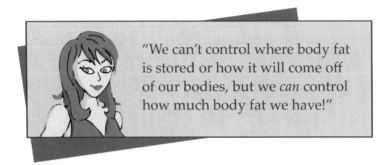

"We can't control where body fat is stored or how it will come off of our bodies, but we *can* control how much body fat we have!"

If your goal is to see your abdominal muscles, reduce cellulite, decrease your waist or hip size, or reduce the "jiggle" on your triceps, you will need to reduce your overall body fat percentage to a level low enough that your body will respond. Doing extra crunches, leg exercises, or tricep kickbacks does NOT reduce body fat in those specific areas—it only tones the muscle under your subcutaneous fat. Your goal of fat loss can only be reached by a complete fat-loss system of proper diet and exercise that will reduce your overall body fat level.

Why do I need to test my body fat periodically?
Knowing your percentage of body fat – and reassessing it periodically – is very useful in gauging progress during an exercise and weight-loss program. It will help guarantee that you are losing fat and gaining muscle. Even if the number on the weight scale doesn't budge, body fat levels will increase over the years when people remain sedentary. So as you age, keeping track of body fat can inspire you to exercise to maintain a healthy ratio of muscle to fat.

How do I get an accurate body fat reading?
There are quite a few methods for measuring body composition, each with its own margin of error, advantages, and disadvantages, as well as special devices, attire, restrictions, and costs.

#1 Underwater Weighing (or Hydrostatic Weighing)

#2 Skin Fold Measurements

#3 Bioelectrical Impedance

#4 Bod Pod (Air Displacement)

#5 Dual Energy X-Ray Absorptiometry (DEXA)

The MY DIVA DIET recommendation is to use the skin fold method, and possibly the Hydrostatic Weighing method, if possible. However, if your body fat level is over 30%, you might consider Bioelectrical Impedance. The most important thing to remember is to use the same method for each test. The skin fold test is subjective, so it is best to visit the same professional for each successive measurement.

How does your body fat compare?
Check your numbers against the standards:
- The Loma Linda University Scale
- The ACE (American Council on Exercise) Scale
- Paw Body Fat Rating Guide (PART THREE, pg. 80 and PART EIGHT, pg. 367)

American Council on Exercise

Classification	Women (% fat)
Essential	10-12%
Athletes	14-20%
Fitness	21-24%
Acceptable	25-31%
Obese	32% +

Loma Linda University
Human Performance Laboratory

Classification	
Lean	<15%
Healthy	15-22%
Plump	23-27%
Fat	28-33%
Obese	33% +

Loma Linda University
Human Performance Laboratory
Continued...

Average middle aged American female = 32%
Average college female = 25%

Athletic Norms

Long distance runners	6-15%
Gymnasts	10-17%
Competitive Bodybuilders	6-10%
Swimmers	14-24%
Basketball athletes	18-27%
Tennis players	19-22%

Diva Worksheet #6
Progress Report

MY Progress Report			
	Starting Point	Week 4	Week 6
Weight (Lb):			
Body Fat (%):			
LBM:			
Fat (Lb):			
Measurements			
Chest (measure at the fullest part of your breasts):			
Waist (measure at the narrowest point above your belly button):			
Abdomen (measure just below your belly button):			
Hips (measure at the widest point around your buttocks):			
Dress Size:			
Pant Size:			
Blouse Size:			
Other (cholesterol, blood pressure, medications, etc.):			
Notes:			

379

MY Progress Report			
	Week 8	Week 10	CHANGES*
Weight (Lb):			
Body Fat (%):			
LBM:			
Fat (Lb):			
Measurements			
Chest (measure at the fullest part of your breasts):			
Waist (measure at the narrowest point above your belly button):			
Abdomen (measure just below your belly button):			
Hips (measure at the widest point around your buttocks):			
Dress Size:			
Pant Size:			
Blouse Size:			
Other (cholesterol, blood pressure, medications, etc.):			
Notes:			

*Compare measurements to your goal sheet (p. 370).

Diva Worksheet #7
3-Week Diet and Exercise Calendar

MY 3-Week Diet & Exercise Calendar				
Week 1	Week of:			
Weekly Weigh-in:				
Day	Diet Today (circle one)	Total Calories	Cheat Day? (circle one)	Exercise Today
Sunday	Good / Great / Poor		Yes / No	
Monday	Good / Great / Poor		Yes / No	
Tuesday	Good / Great / Poor		Yes / No	
Wednesday	Good / Great / Poor		Yes / No	
Thursday	Good / Great / Poor		Yes / No	
Friday	Good / Great / Poor		Yes / No	
Saturday	Good / Great / Poor		Yes / No	
Notes:				

MY 3-Week Diet & Exercise Calendar				
Week 2	Week of:			
Weekly Weigh-in:				
Day	Diet Today (circle one)	Total Calories	Cheat Day? (circle one)	Exercise Today
Sunday	Good / Great / Poor		Yes / No	
Monday	Good / Great / Poor		Yes / No	
Tuesday	Good / Great / Poor		Yes / No	
Wednesday	Good / Great / Poor		Yes / No	
Thursday	Good / Great / Poor		Yes / No	
Friday	Good / Great / Poor		Yes / No	
Saturday	Good / Great / Poor		Yes / No	
Notes:				

MY 3-Week Diet & Exercise Calendar				
Week 3	Week of:			
Weekly Weigh-in:				
Day	Diet Today (circle one)	Total Calories	Cheat Day? (circle one)	Exercise Today
Sunday	Good / Great / Poor		Yes / No	
Monday	Good / Great / Poor		Yes / No	
Tuesday	Good / Great / Poor		Yes / No	
Wednesday	Good / Great / Poor		Yes / No	
Thursday	Good / Great / Poor		Yes / No	
Friday	Good / Great / Poor		Yes / No	
Saturday	Good / Great / Poor		Yes / No	
Notes:				

Diva Worksheet #8
MY DIVA DIET Journal

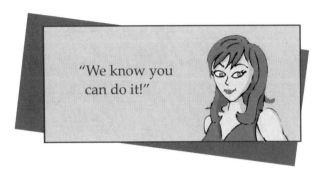

"We know you can do it!"

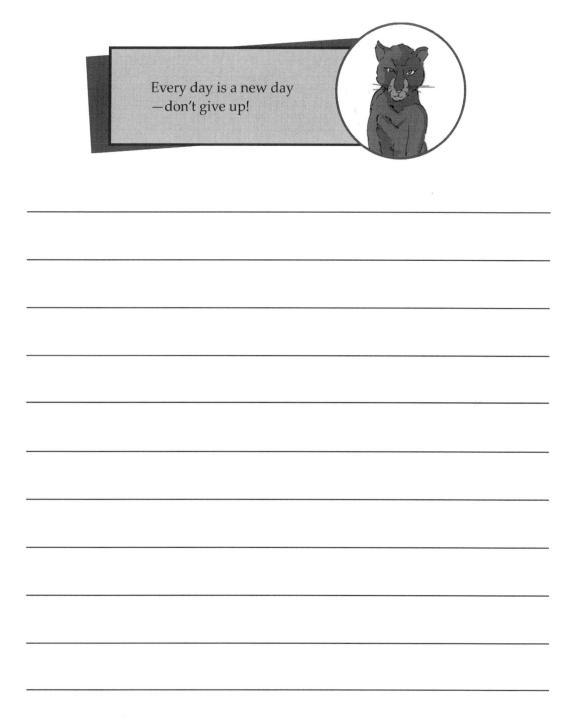

Every day is a new day
—don't give up!

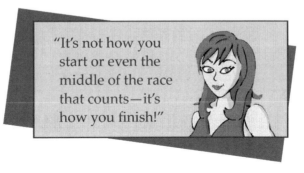

"It's not how you start or even the middle of the race that counts—it's how you finish!"

MY DIVA DIET Resource & Recommendations

MY DIVA DIET was built around twenty-five years in the fitness industry, thirteen years of health & fitness education, and over ten years of research. Our experience is not only in helping others, but also in applying it to our own personal lives!

We used our resources to help build a great diet program. We also used them to confirm some of our information and to dig deeper into particular topics. We wanted to make sure that we explained things completely and accurately. We even looked at resources to see the other side of our arguments.

Even though we at MY DIVA DIET have extensive backgrounds in the fitness industry and are known for helping thousands lose fat and increase health, we feel that we are NOT the only fat-loss program based on sound nutrition, and results. There are programs that will enhance ours, especially those with great recipe ideas. The diet industry is a $50 billion dollar-a-year business, which means there are too many books, programs and websites to choose from. We want to help you check into other programs, books, websites, and other pertinent information.

We also want you to be as informed as possible so that you will not deviate from our healthy fat-loss program or others you might try. As you become more grounded in your lifestyle of proper dieting and exercise, you will be able to spot any gimmick that comes along the way! Our goal is that our diet book will be the "Last Diet Book" you will ever need, and our mission is to ensure that you will attain a lean, healthy, fit, and more functional body—for life!

Fitness, Health & Medical Organizations

ACE American Council on Exercise. <http://www.acefitness.org>.

American Heart Association. <http://www.americanheart.org>.

Chek, Paul. The Chek Institute. <http://www.chekinstitute.com>.

Colbert, Dr. Don. Dr. Don Colbert. <http://www.drcolbert.com>.

John Hopkins Bayview Medical Center. <http://www.jhbmc.jhu.edu>.

Loma Linda University. <http://www.llu.edu>.

National Institute of Diabetes and Digestive and Kidney Disorders.
    <http://www2.niddk.nih.gov>.

NESTA National Exercise & Sports Trainers Association.
    <http://www.nestacertified.com>.

WEB MD. <http://www.webmd.com>.

Books, Websites & Films To Consider
Books:

Balch, Phyllis A., C.N.C., and James F. Balch, M.D. Nutritional Healing. New York,
    NY: Avery, 2002.

Bricklin, Mark. Prevention Magazine's Nutrition Advisor. Emmaus, PA: Rodale
    Press, Inc., 1993.

Chek, Paul. How to Eat, Move and Be Healthy. San Diego, CA: C.H.E.K Institute,
    2004. <http://www.chekinstitute.com>.

Cloutier, Marissa, M.S. R.D., and Eve Adamson. The Mediterranean Diet. New York,
    NY: Harper Collins Publishers, 2001.

Colbert, Don. <u>What Would Jesus Eat?</u> (Book and cookbook). Nashville, TN: Thomas Nelson Publishers, 2002.

Colbert, Don. <u>The Seven Pillars of Health.</u> Lake Mary: Siloam Press, 2007.

Cruise, Jorge. <u>The 3-Hour Diet.</u> New York, NY: Harper Collins Publishers, 2007 <http://www.3hourdiet.com>.

Freedman, Rory, and Barnouin, Kim. <u>Skinny Bitch.</u> Philadelphia, PA: Running Press Book Publishers, 2005. <http://www.skinnybitch.net>.

Gittleman, Anne Louise, Ph. D. <u>The Fat Flush Plan.</u> New York, NY: McGraw-Hill, 2002. <http://www.annlouise.com>.

Greene, Bob. <u>The Best Life Diet.</u> New York, NY: Simon & Schuster, 2006. <http://www.bestlifediet.com>.

Kirschmann, Gayla J., and John D. Kirschmann. <u>Nutrition Almanac Fourth Edition.</u> New York, NY: McGraw-Hill, 1996.

Mateljan, George. <u>The World's Healthiest Foods.</u> Seattle, WA: George Mateljan Foundation, 2007. <http://www.whfoods.com>.

Rena, Tosca, B.Sc.,B.Ed. <u>The Eat Clean Diet</u> (Book and cookbook). Mississauga, Ontario, Canada: Robert Kennedy, 2007 <http://www.eatcleandiet.com>.

Rodriguez, Judith C., Ph.D., R.D., F.A.D.A. <u>The Diet Selector.</u> Philadelphia, PA: Running Press Book Publishers, 2007. <http://www.runningpresscooks.com>.

Rubin, Jordan S. <u>The Maker's Diet.</u> New York, NY: The Berkley Publishing Group, 2004. <http://www.themakersdiet.com>.

Schlosser, Eric. <u>Fast Food Nation.</u> New York, NY: Harper Collins Publishers, 2001.

Young, Robert O., Ph.D., and Shelley Redford Young. <u>The pH Miracle.</u> New York, NY: Warner Books, Inc., 2002.

Films:
<u>Fast Food Nation.</u> Dir. Richard Linklater. Film. 2006.

<u>Supersize Me.</u> Dir. Morgan Spurlock. Film. 2004.

Websites:
<u>BodyBuilding.com</u> <http://www.bodybuilding.com>.

<u>Fit Day.</u> <http://www.fitday.com>.

Mercola, Dr. Joseph. <u>Dr. Joseph Mercola.</u> <http://www.mercola.com>.

Michaels, Jillian. <u>Losing It with Jillian Michaels.</u> <http://www.jillianmichaels.com>.

<u>Nutrimundo Diet, The.</u> <http://www.nutrimundo.com>.

<u>Shape Fit.</u> <shapefit.com>.

Nutrition Calculators & Food Value Information
<u>Calorie Count.</u> <http://www.calorie-count.com>.

<u>Calorie King.</u> <http://www.calorieking.com>.

<u>The Calorie Counter.</u> <http://www.thecaloriecounter.com>.

Netzer, Corrine. <u>The Corinne T. Netzer Encyclopedia of Food Values.</u> New York: Dell Publishing, 1992.

<u>Nut Nutrition.</u> <http://www.nutnutrition.com>.

Nutrition Data. <http://www.nutritiondata.com>.

Whole Foods Market. <http://www.wholefoodsmarket.com>.

Recommended Food Companies & Products & Supermarkets
Amy's. <http://www.amys.com>.

Ancient Foods. <http://www.ancientharvest.com>.

Annie's Naturals. <http://www.consorzio.com>.

Applegate Farms. <http://www.applegatefarms.com>.

Arrowhead Mills. <http://www.arrowheadmills.com>.

Bakery on Main Gourmet Naturals. <http://www.bakeryonmain.com>.

Boar's Head. <http://www.boarshead.com>.

Bolthouse Farms. <http://www.bolthouse.com>.

Dole. <http://www.dole.com>.

Edamame. <http://www.localharvest.org

Eden Organic. <http://www.edenfoods.com>.

Erewhon Natural Foods Market. <http://www.erewhonmarket.com>.

Fantastic World Foods. <http://www.fantasticfoods.com>.

Food For Life. <http://www.foodforlife.com>.

French Meadow Bakery Organic Products. <http://www.frenchmeadow.com>.

Gluten Free Foods. <http://www.glutenfree.com>.

Gluten Smart. <http://www.glutensmart.com>.

Gold Mine Natural Foods. <http://www.goldminenaturalfood.com>.

Grainaissance. <http://www.grainaissance.com>.

Guiltless Gourmet. <http://www.guiltlessgourmet.com>.

Health Valley. <http://www.healthvalley.com>.

Hebrew National. <http://www.hebrewnational.com>.

Heidi's Hens. <http://www.diestelturkey.com>.

Honey Gardens. <http://www.honeygardens.com>.

Horizon Organic. <http://www.horizonorganic.com>.

Imagine Organic Gourmet Soups. <http://www.imaginefoods.com>.

Julian Bakery. <http://www.julianbakery.net>.

Kashi Products. <http://www.kashi.com>.

Kosher foods. <http://aaronsgourmet.pagedepot.com>.

Living Fuel. <http://www.livingfuel.com>.

Lotus Foods. (grains and legumes) <http://www.worldpantry.com>.

Lundberg Family Farms, since 1937. <http://www.lundberg.com>.

MaraNatha. <http://www.worldpantry.com>.

Melissa's. <http://www.melissas.com>.

Mexi-Snax. <http://www.mexisnax.com>.

Muir Glen Organic. <http://www.muirglen.com>.

Nancy's Springfield Creamery. <http://www.nancysyogurt.com>.

Nasoya. <http://www.nasoya.com>.

Nu-World Foods. <http://www.nuworldamaranth.com>.

Organic Valley. <http://www.organicvalley.com>.

Pacific Natural Foods. <http://www.pacificfoods.com>.

Que Pasa Mexican Foods. <http://www.quepasafoods.com>.

Quinoa Corporation. <http://www.quinoa.net>.

Real Foods. <http://www.cornthins.com>.

Rising Moon Organics. <http://www.risingmoon.com>.

San-J. <http://www.san-j.com>.

Santa Cruz Organic. <http://www.scojuice.com>.

Seeds Of Change. <http://www.seedsofchangefoods.com>.

Simply Organic. <http://www.simplyorganicfoods.com>.

Sno Pac Organic. <http://www.snopac.com>.

Spectrum. <http://www.spectrumorganics.com>.

Stonyfield Organic Farm. <http://www.stonyfield.com>.

Sunnyside Farms. <http://www.sunnysideorganic.com>.

SunRidge Farms. <http://www.sunridgefarms.com>.

The World's Healthiest Foods. <http://www.whfoods.org>.

The Whole Wheatery. <http://www.thewholewheatery.com>.

Tinkyada. <http://www.tinkyada.com>.

Trader Joes Grocery Store. <http://www.traderjoes.com>.

Tropical Traditions. <http://www.tropicaltraditions.com>.

Vital Choice Wild Seafood & Organics. <http://www.vitalchoice.com>.

WestBrae Natural. <http://www.westbrae.com>.

Whole Foods Market. <http://www.wholefoodsmarket.com>.

Wild Harvest Organic. <http://www.wildharvest.com>.

Wilderness Family Naturals. <http://www.wildernessfamilynaturals.com>.

Resources

Section Pages of MY DIVA DIET:
"Women's History (Quotations by Notable Women)." About.com.
   <http://womenshistory.about.com/library/qu/blqulist.htm>.

Statistics on Dieting & Food Disorders:
Alfonsi, Sharyn. "Diet Industry Is Big Business." CBS News. December 1, 2006.

Calorie Control Council. <caloriecontrol.org>.

Goodstein, Ellen. "10 Secrets of the Weight-loss Industry." Bankrate.com.
   <http://www.bankrate.com>.

HealthyWithin.com. "Statistics and Pre-Signs of Eating Disorders."
   <http://www.healthywithin.com>.

INCH-A-WEIGH.com. <http://www.inch-a-weigh.com>.

NEDIC (National Eating Disorder Information Centre) News.
   <http://www.nedic.ca>.

Penn State University Health Services. < www.sa.psu.edu/uhs/>.

Food Labels, Food Safety & Food Additives:
"Deciphering Food Labels." Kid's Health.org.
   <http://www.kidshealth.org/parent/nutrition_fit/nutrition/food_labels.html>.

"Food Safety and Food Additives." Center for Science in the Public Interest.
   <http://www.cspinet.org>.

"List of Food Additives." Wikipedia Free Encyclopedia.
   <http://www.wikipedia.org>.

Organic Information:

Benbrook, Charles, Preston Andrews, Neal Davies, Jaime Yanez, and Xin Zhao. "New Evidence Confirms the Nutritional Superiority of Plant-Based Organic Foods." The Organic Center State of Science Review: Nutritional Superiority of Organic Foods. March 2008 <http://www.organic-center.org>.

Burros, Marian. "Is Organic Food More Nutritious?" The New York Times. July 2003. Organic Consumer Association. <http://www.organicconsumers.org>.

Compassion Over Killing. <http://www.cok.net>.

Dauncey, Guy. "Ten Reasons Why Organic Food is Better." Earth Future Earth. August 2002. <http://www.earthfuture.com/earth/>.

Mercola, Dr. Joseph. "It's Official: Organic Really is Better." Mercola.com. <http://articles.mercola.com/sites/articles/archive/2007/11/17/it-s-official-organic-really-is-better.aspx>.

Leahy, Stephen. "New Studies Back Benefits of Organic Diet." CommonDreams.Org News Center. 4 March 2006. <http://www.commondreams.org>.

"Organic Diets Lower Children's Dietary Exposure to Common Agriculture Pesticides." Emory University Research Study. 2006. <http://www.emory.edu>.

"Organic Food." Wikipedia Free Encyclopedia. <http://www.wikipedia.org>.

"Organically Grown Foods Higher In Cancer-Fighting Chemicals Than Conventionally Grown Foods." Science Daily. 4 March 2003. <http://www.sciencedaily.com>.

"The Organic Myth." Business Week Magazine Online. <http://www.businessweek.com>.

Ungoed-Thomas, Jon. "Eat Your Words, All Who Scoff at Organic Food." Times Online. 28 October 2007. <http://www.timesonline.co.uk>.

Other Resources:

Better Health Channel. <http://www.betterhealth.vic.gov.au>.

Celiac Disease Foundation. <http://www.celiac.org>.

Dairy Council of California. <http://www.dairycouncilofca.org>.

Foundation of Wellness. <http://www.wellnessletter.com>.

Fruit and Veggies More Matters Organization.
   <http://www.fruitsandveggiesmorematters.org>.

Gluten Intolerance and Celiac Disease - The Food Intolerance Consumer.
   <http://www.foodintol.com>.

HealthCastle.com. <http://www.healthcastle.com>./nutrition

Health Check Systems. <http://www.healthchecksystems.com>.

Health Line. <http://www.healthline.com>.

"Human Nutrition, Foods, and Exercise." Virginia Tech University.
   <http://www.virginiatech.com>.

Jay's Information. <http://www.tripod.com>.

Judaism 101 Dietary Laws. <http://www.jewfaq.org>.

Kosher Triangle. <http://www.hebrewnational.com>.

National Dairy Council. <http://www.nationaldairycouncil.org>.

Natural Zing Market. <http://www.naturalzing.com>.

Pure Zing. <http://www.purezing.com>.

Raw Food Life. <http://www.rawfoodlife.com>.

RecipeTips.com. <http://www.recipetips.com>.

Shape Fit. <http://www.shapefit.com>.

Sprout People. <http://www.sproutpeople.com>.

The Breadery. <http://www.thebreadery.com>.

The Gluten Free Mall. <http://www.theglutenfreemall.com>.

Wikipedia Free Encyclopedia. <http://www.wikipedia.org>

Miscellaneous Websites & Articles
Coffee & Tea:
HealthCastle.com. <http://www.healthcastle.com/tea.shtml>.

Starbucks. <http://www.starbucks.com>.

Dairy:
Barrett, Stephen, M.D. "Why Raw Milk Should be Avoided." Quack Watch.com.
    <http://www.quackwatch.com>.

Bunton, Molly. "Info on Raw Milk & Pasturization." Fias Co. Farm.
    <http://fiascofarm.com/dairy/rawmilk.htm#pasteurization>.

"Got Milk? Make Sure It's Pasteurized." U.S. Food and Drug Administration Consumer
    Magazine. 2004. <http://www.fda.gov/fdac/features/2004/504_milk.html>.

Schmidt, Ron, N.D. "Health Benefits of Raw Milk From Grass-Fed Animals."
  <http://www.realmilk.com/healthbenefits.html>.

"The Health Benefits of Raw Milk." White Tiger Productions. 2007
  <http://www.raw-milk-facts.com/raw_milk_health_benefits.html>.

Fast Food Information:
Baja Fresh. <http://www.bajafresh.com>.

Burger King. <http://www.burgerking.com>.

Carl's Jr. <http://www.carlsjr.com>.

Dairy Queen. <http://www.dairyqueen.com>.

Hardee's. <http://www.hardees.com>.

Jack n the Box. <http://www.jackinthebox.com>.

Kentucky Fried Chicken. <http://www.kfc.com>.

Long John Silver's. <http://www.ljsilvers.com>.

McDonalds. <http://www.mcdonalds.com>.

Panda Express. <http://www.pandaexpress.com>.

Quiznos. <http://www.quiznos.com>.

Round Table Pizza. <http://www.roundtablepizza.com>.

Sonic. <http://www.sonicdrivein.com>.

Subway. <http://www.subway.com>.

Taco Bell. <http://www.tacobell.com>.

Wendy's. <http://www.wendys.com>.

Whataburger. <http://www.whataburger.com>.

Protein Powders & Supplements:
Energy First ProEnergy Whey Protein Powder. <http://www.energyfirst.com>.

GeniSoy Natural Protein Powder. <http://www.drugstore.com>.

Jay Robb Protein Powders and Bars. <http://www.jayrobb.com>.

National Institute of Health – Office of Dietary Supplements.
   <http://dietary-supplements.info.nih.gov/>.

Nutiva Organic Hemp Protein Powder. <http://www.globalhempstore.com>.

Oregon State University. Linus Pauling Institute
   <http://www.oregonstateuniversity.com>.

Solaray Supplements. <http://www.affordablesolaray.com>.

VitaminDeals.com. <http://www.vitamindeals.com>.

Vitamins & Supplements Guide. <http://www.vitamins-supplements.org>.

World's Healthiest Foods. <http://www.whfoods.com>.

Zest for Life. <http://www.anyvitamins.com>.

Vitamin & Mineral Articles:

 At the Family Place – Acidophilus. <http://www.atthefamilyplace.com/acidopholus-bacteria-aids-a-culture-of-digestion>.

"Calcium." Better Health Channel. 2007. <http://wwwbetterhealth.vic.gov.au/BHCV2?bhcarticles.nsf/pages/Calcium?OpenDocument>.

Doctor Yourself. <http://www.doctoryourself.com>.

Mangels, Reed, Ph.D., R.D. "Calcium in the Vegan Diet." The Vegan Resource Group Nutrition. 2006. <http://www.vrg.org/nutrition/calcium.htm#table1>.

Vitamin and Nutrition Center. <http://www.vitamins-nutrition.org>.

Water:

Don Colbert, M.D. <http://www.drcolbert.com>.

Mayo Clinic. <http://www.MayoClinic.com>.

U.S Food and Drug Administration. <http://www.fda.gov>.

Miscellaneous Articles:

"Alcohol and Health." Bristol.org. <http://www.at-bristol.org.uk/Alcoholandyou/Society/health.html>.

Alden, Lori. "Grain Products Category (1996-2005)." The Cook's Thesaurus. <http://www.foodsubs.comFGGrainProd.html>.

"All About Chocolate: The History of Chocolate." The Field Museum. 2007. <http://www.fieldmuseum.org/Chocolate/history.html>.

"Americans Are Obsessed with Fast Food: The Dark Side." CBS News Interview With
Schlosser, Eric. CBS News.
<http://www.cbsnews.com/stories/2002/01/31health/main326858.shtml>.

Anderson, J., S. Perryman, L. Young. "Understanding the Food Label." Colorado
State University. 2007. <http://www.extcolostate.edu/pubs/foodnut/09365.html>.

Armstrong, Eric. "What's Wrong with Partially Hydrogenated Oils?"
Tree Light Store. 2001, 2005, 2007.
<http://www.treelight.com/health/nutrition/PartiallyHydrogenatedOils.html>.

"Basic Egg Facts." The American Egg Board.
<http://www.aeb.org/LearnMore/EggFacts.htm>.

Bell, Brenda. "Can you explain the terms 'whole grain' and 'stone ground'?"
Missouri Families; University of Missouri Extension - Food and Fitness. 2001.
<http://missourifamilies.org/quick/nutritionqa/nutqa69.htm>.

Calzadilla, Raphael, B.A., CPT. "Cellulite Cures – The Truths." E-Diets.com.
<http://www.ediets.com/news/printArticle.cfm?cid=1&cmi=1976820>.

"Celiac Disease." NDDIC - National Digestive Disease Information Clearinghouse.
<http://digestive.niddk.nih.gov/ddiseases/pubs/celiac/>.

Challem, Jack. "Fructose Maybe Not So Natural… and Not So Safe." The Nutrition
Reporter. <http://www.thenutritionreporter.com/fructose_dangers.html>.

Chang, Louise, M.D. (reviewer). "Eggs: Dietary Friend of Foe." Web MD Health &
Diet. 2006. <http://www.webmd.com/diet/features/eggs-dietary-friend-foe>.

Chocolate Necessities Nutritional Information 2001-2008.
<http://www.chocolatenecessities.com>.

Collins, Anne. "Good Fats to Eat (2000-2007)" AnneCollins.com.
  <http://www.annecollins.com/good-fats-to-eat.htm>.

"Constipation." NDDIC - National Digestive Disease Information Clearinghouse.
  <http://digestive.niddk.nih.gov/ddiseases/pubs/constipation/>.

Dolson, Laura. "Fructose Sweet, But Dangerous." 2007.
  <http://lowcarbdiets.about.com/od/nutrition/a/fructosedangers.htm?p=1>.

Dowshen, Steven, M.D. (reviewer). "What is Cellulite?"
  Nemours Foundation Teens Health. 2006.
  <http://www.kidshealth.org/teen/your_body/beautiful/cellulite.html

"Guidelines for Optimal Health." Living Fuel. 2005.
  <http://www.livingfuel.com/GON.htm>.

"How do honey bees make honey? What is honey?" CoolQuiz.com.
  <http://www.coolquiz.com>.

Jones, Susan, Ph.D. "Sweat Your Way To Radiant Health." Eco Mail.
  <http://www.ecomall.com>./greenshopping/sauna1.htm>.

"Know Your Fats." American Heart Association. 2008.
  <http://www.americanheart.org>.

Kryzanowski, Paul. "Potted Meat Food Products." PK.org.
  <http://www.pk.org/pottedmeat.html>.

Leduc, Marc. "Sugar's effect on your health." HealingDaily.com. 2007.
  <http://www.healingdaily.com/detoxification-diet/sugar.htm>.

Mercola, Dr. Joseph. "Fat, $100 Billion Crisis." Mercola.com. 2007.
  <http://articles.mercola.com/sites/articles/archive/2007/09/29/a-fat-100-billion-crisis.aspx>.

"Rice Cake." How Products Are Made - Volume 4.
   <http://www.madehow.com>./Volume-4/Rice-Cake.html>.

Roubos, Dane A., D.C. "The Margarine Hoax." 1997.
   <http://www.drcranton.com/nutrition/margarin.htm>.

Sands, Bill, BS, MBA. "The Double Danger of High Fructose Corn Syrup."
   The Weston A. Price Foundation. 2003.
   <http://www.westonaprice.org/modernfood/highfructose.html>.

"Sugar Sweet By Nature." Sugar.com. <http://www.sugar.org>.

"Sugar Effects on Your Health." HealingDaily.com. 2007.
   <http://www.healingdialy.com>./detoxification-diet/sugar.htm

"The Dangers of Meat." PBS Frontline Documentary. 2002.
   <http://www.stephen-knapp.com/the_dangers_of_meat.htm>.

"The History of Popcorn." Essortment Information. 2002.
   <http://okok.essortment.com/whatisthehist_rsdt.htm>.

"The Mediterranean Diet." American Heart Association. 2008
   <http://www.americanheart.org/presenter.jhtml?identifier=4644>.

"Water: How Much Should You Drink Every Day?" Mayo Clinic. CNN.com Health
   Library. <http://www.cnn.com/health/library/NU/00283.html>.

"What Color is Your Food? Plant Pigments For Color and Nutrition."
   University of Wisconsin.
   <http://www.hort.wisc.edu/usdavcru/simon/publications/97hort0012.html>.

"What is Hummus?" WiseGeek.com.
   <http://www.wisegeek.com/what-is-hummus.htm>.

"What is Molasses?" <u>WiseGeek.com.</u>
   <http://www.wisegeek.com/what-is-molasses.htm>.

"Wheat - The Inside Story." <u>Library Think Quest.</u>
   <http://library.thinkquest.org/11226/main/c02.htm>.

"Why is it important to eat grains, especially whole grains?" <u>United States Department of Agriculture.</u> <http://www.mypyramid.gov/pyramid/grains_why_print.html>

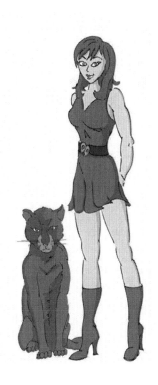

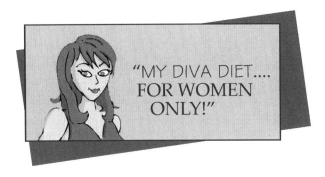

Christine Lakatos, creator of the MY DIVA DIET fat-loss system and workbook, has been involved in the health & fitness industry since 1980, and has been a personal fitness consultant and trainer since 1989. ACE certified since 1995, she has studied scientific back training, program design, Swiss ball training, rehabilitation training, scientific core conditioning, strength training for women, maternal and infant nutrition, childhood and adolescent nutrition, and weight management for teens, plus much more.

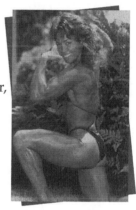

Her journey in the field of fitness began in early childhood when she was a "track star", and resumed later as an adult when she became a competitor in both bodybuilding and fitness. It quickly progressed to her becoming a teacher, coaching and helping others to get fit. After retiring as a fitness competitor, her fascination for nutrition became her new mission, and she studied it from every angle possible. As a result of her competition days, her ability to get her own body fat to 6%, and her aptitude to maintain between 12-15% body fat in her adult life (done naturally, without starving or drugs), she wanted to share this great news with other women. Since 1990 she has shared this knowledge with thousands of her clients, and all who followed the plan not only lost fat but also improved their health dramatically.

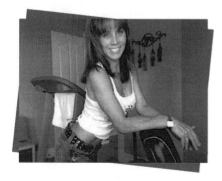

Now in her forties, Christine strives to make sure women understand that there is no quick-fix to fat loss, improving health, and increasing longevity, and that dieting to lose weight is not about deprivation. She teaches that the key to fat loss and vibrant health is accomplished through a lifestyle change by means of accountability, discipline, and motivation.

Her specific goal in developing MY DIVA DIET is to empower women to adopt proper eating habits and effective exercise programs—that will not only help them look better, but will cause them to feel and function better, **challenging them to be better women**—for life! The mother of two wonderful children, Christine knows that you can have low body fat and great health in your youth and adult years, even after having and raising children!

Christine has won titles in many competitions: 1993 Ms. Fitness San Diego, 1990 Ms. Fitness USA—Top 10 finalist, 1990 Steel Rose Championship finalist, and 1989 Ms. San Luis Obispo. She has also made promotional appearances for the health & fitness industry for: Thane Fitness Co., Power Gym, KESQ TV 3 Midday Show, Muscle Mag Video, Joe Weider's Muscle & Fitness camp (counselor), Parillo Performance, Strong & Shapely, and Ironman magazine. She was also an American Gladiators (1990) contestant.

Amber Garman has a passion for health, nutrition, and fitness. As a young woman in a wheelchair, she particularly understands that learning about proper nutrition is fundamental to health and well-being. She loves learning about all aspects of the health field, especially cooking, and is always continuing her education in this area. Amber, also an avid exerciser, knows firsthand the value of what a good diet and an exercise program can do for you physically, emotionally, and mentally.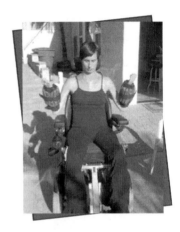

After being paralyzed in a car accident, Amber soon realized her body no longer worked and functioned the same way it had before. With no instruction manual coming with her injury, she began experimenting with all sorts of healthy ingredients, herbs, and ways of cooking and pairing foods. She soon discovered that her body was functioning with ease, had a much higher level of energy, and her overall appearance was brighter and healthier looking. The dramatic difference Amber saw and felt between her new diet and her old diet was and is a substantial lifestyle upgrade.

In finding the beneficial results with changing her diet and adding a stretching and weight-lifting program, Amber would like to make a special note to other handicapped and disabled women about MY DIVA DIET if you are interested in losing weight and gaining health while being handicapped or disabled, this program will work for you. Also, on the other side of the spectrum, are people like Amber, who are trying to gain and maintain their weight—MY DIVA DIET **will** work for you. Having a healthy diet and exercise program is a must for women who are handicapped and disabled—you will never go back to your old unhealthy eating habits!

It was a perfect match for Amber and her Aunt Christine to write this book together so that these two "health-inspired" people could help inspire others. MY DIVA DIET can help not only women who are able-bodied, but our program can also help disabled women, which is truly important to Amber.

Amber is currently completing an A.A. degree in general studies and continuing independent health research, which she started five years ago. She has participated in and taught special techniques of physical therapy developed by Aaron Mattes, M.S., R.K.T., L.K.T., including Active Isolated Stretching.

MY DIVA DIET Directory
Special Superhero Designs, Paw Guides &
MY DIVA DIET Guides

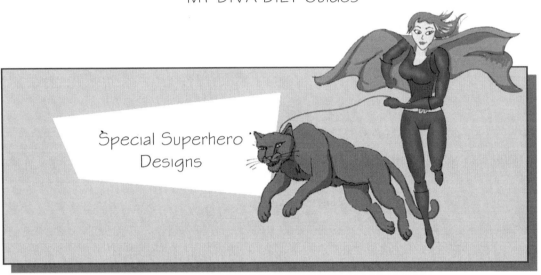

Special Superhero Designs

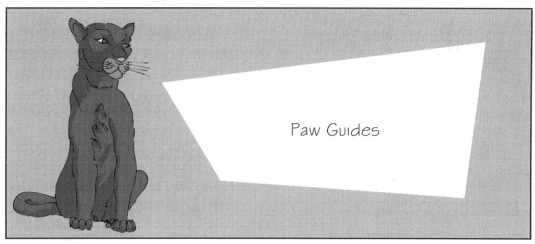

Paw Guides

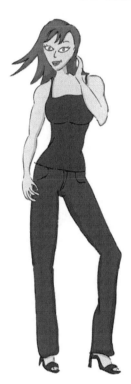

MY DIVA DIET Guides

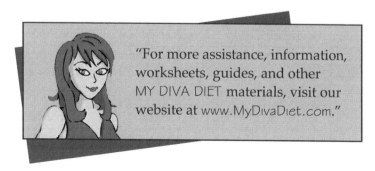

"For more assistance, information, worksheets, guides, and other MY DIVA DIET materials, visit our website at www.MyDivaDiet.com."

2854748